Keto Diet

The Ultimate Ketogenic Diet Cookbook Guide for Weight Loss, Delicious and Easy Recipes

Additionally, the information in the following pages is intended only for informational purposes and should thus be thought of as universal. As befitting its nature, it is presented without assurance regarding its prolonged validity or interim quality. Trademarks that are mentioned are done without written consent and can in no way be considered an endorsement from the trademark holder.

Table of Contents

KETO CHOCOLATE MOUSSE 9

KETO CHOCOLATE CAKE WITH WHIPPED CREAM ICING 11

KETO BROWNIES 13

NO BAKE KETO CHEESECAKE FLUFF 15

KETO CHOCOLATE CHIP COOKIES 17

KETO MUG CAKE 19

KETO LOW CARB BLUEBERRY CRISPS 21

SUGAR FREE CHOCOLATE BARK WITH BACON AND ALMONDS 23

KETO BROWN BUTTER PRALINES 25

THE BEST KETO CHEESECAKE 27

KETO CHICKEN AND BROCCOLI CASSEROLE 30

KETO BBQ RIBS 32

KETO SHRIMPS SCAMPI 35

LOW CARBS BACON CHEESE CASSEROLE 37

KETO CHICKEN BREAST POT PIE WITH CAULIFLOWER CRUST 39

KETO SPINACH ARTICHOK 42

KETO LEMON GARLIC CHICKEN THIGHS IN THE AIR FRYER 44

KETO MEATBALLS 46

KETO FRIENDLY SOUP 49

KETO FRIENDLY BARBECUED BANANA PRAWNS 51

KETO FRIENDLY CREAMY AVOCADO ZOODLES 53

BAKED SAUSAGE RATATOUILLE 55

KETO FRIENDLY SALMON WITH TAHINI DRESSING 57

KETO FRIENDLY TUNA POKE BOWL 59

KETO CHICKEN CURRY WITH TURMERIC RICE 62

BAKED SALMON FILLET WITH RAW BROCCOLI SALAD 64

KETO FRIENDLY LAMB TAGINE 66

KETO FRIENDLY 20-MINUTES CHICKEN 68

KETO FRIENDLY ZOODLES AND EGG SALAD 70

KETO GROUND CHICKEN TACOS 72

KETO PIZZA ROLL UPS 74

KETO CAULIFLOWER MAC AND CHEESE 76

KETO SPINACH ARTICHOKE DIP 78

KETO SAUSAGE PIZZA BITES 81

KETO STUFFED MUSHROOMS 83

KETO ASPARAGUS FRIES 85

KETO CHEESE STUFFED MEATBALLS 88

KETO BACON WRAPPED BRUSSELS SPROUTS 90

KETO TURKEY BACON RANCH PINWHEELS 92

SMOKED TROUT MOUSSE 94

SHRIMP RANGOON MINI BELL PEPPERS APPETIZER 96

KETO CRANBERRY BRIE BITES 98

KETO BACON, EGG AND CHEESE SLIDER APPETIZER 100

KETO RANCH DIP 102

KETO SHRIMP AVOCADO CUCUMBER BITES... 104

SALAMI APPETIZERS 106

KETO SHRIMP GUACAMOLE 108

KETO CRANBERRY MEATBALLS 110

SOUR CREAM AND ONION KETO CHIPS... 112

KETO ZUCCHINI PIZZA CRUST.. 114

NOTES 118

Recipe No 1

Keto Chocolate Mousse

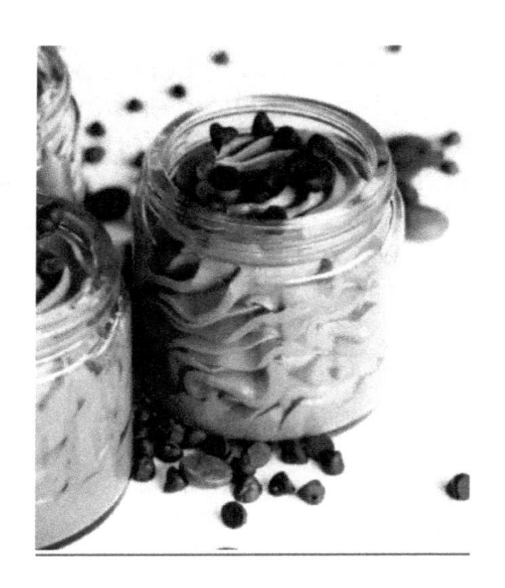

Preparing Time: 15 minutes,
Cooking Time: 5minutes
Serving: 2 people

Ingredients

- 2 cups of heavy whipping cream
- ¼ cup of cocoa powder
- 1 tablespoon of stevia sweetener
- Dark chocolate chips for toppings

Directions

- Take an electric hand mixer and bowl
- Add heavy whipping cream, cocoa powder, stevia sweetener, mix then and converts into smooth mixture and make thick and stiff peaks formed
- Take a piping bag and add the chocolate mousse and pour it into the jar. Top with the chocolate chip and enjoy

Recipe No 2

Keto Chocolate Cake With Whipped Cream Icing

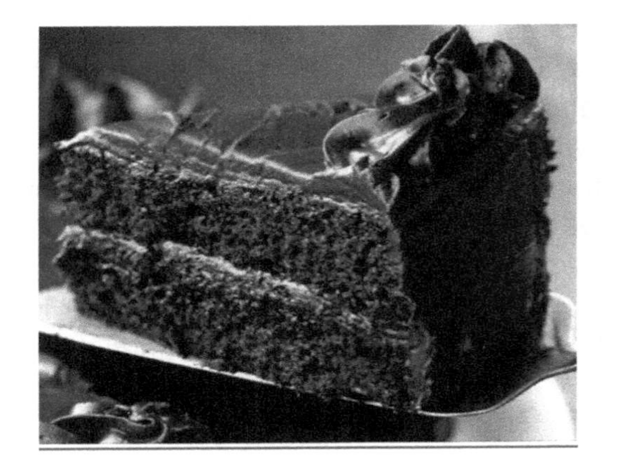

Preparing Time: 15 minutes,
Cooking Time: 35 minutes
Serving: 4 people

Ingredients

- 2 cups of almond flour
- ¼ cup of cocoa powder
- 2 tablespoons of Dutch cocoa powder
- 2 tablespoons of baking powder
- Pinch of salt to taste
- ⅓ cup of almond milk
- 3 golden eggs
- ⅓ cup of granulated sugar
- 2 tablespoons of vanilla extract

Directions

- Preheat the oven at 180 F lined with parchment paper
- Take a bowl add all the ingredients together and blend them with an electric hand mixer
- Pour the batter in the baking 8 inches deep pan and let them bake for about 15 minutes. Remove from the oven and let them cool
- Spread the dark melted chocolate and refrigerate the for about 30 minutes and serve chilled

Recipe No 3

Keto Brownies

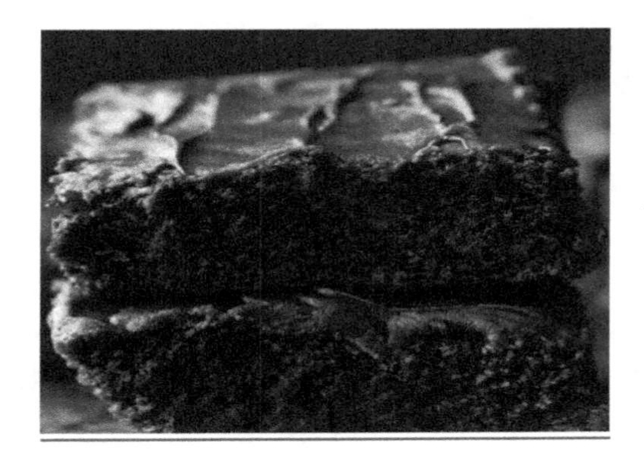

Preparing Time: 10 minutes,
Cooking Time: 25 minutes
Serving: 4 people

Ingredients

- 2 cups of almond flour
- 3 tablespoons of cocoa powder
- 2 tablespoons of Dutch cocoa powder
- Pinch of salt to taste
- ½ teaspoon of baking powder
- 3 tablespoon of coconut oil
- 3 tablespoons of water
- 2 golden eggs
- 2 cups of granulated sugar
- 1 teaspoon of vanilla extract

Directions

- Preheat the oven at 180 F
- Take a baking pan of about 8 inches lined with the parchment paper and greased with almond oil
- Take a bowl add all the ingredients together and mix them by using electric hand mixer
- Pour this batter in the pan and line the parchment paper on the top and bake them for about 20 minutes
- After 20 minutes remove them from the oven and let them cool down remove the parchment paper and spread melted dark chocolate on the top
- Put them in the refrigerator for about 1 hour after 1 hour remove them and cut them into pieces and serve
- Enjoy

Recipe No 4

No Bake Keto Cheesecake Fluff

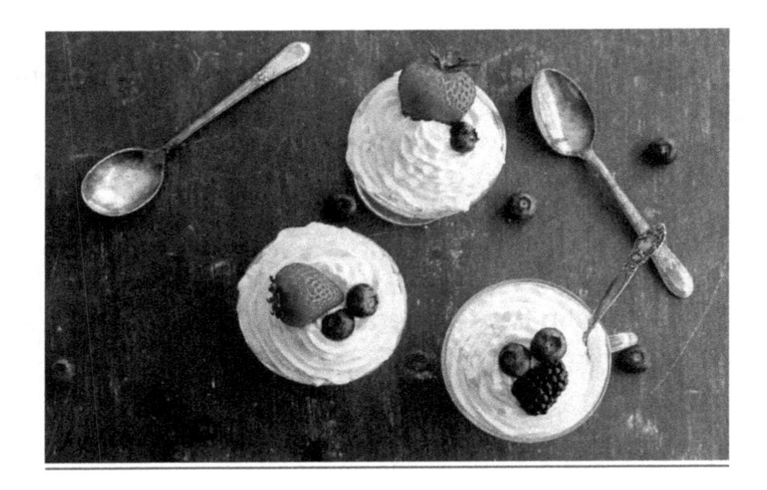

Preparing Time: 10 minutes,
Cooking Time: 35 minutes
Serving: 5 people

Ingredients

- 2 cups of cream cheese
- 1 cup of heavy whipping cream
- ¼ cup of sweetener
- Some blueberries and strawberries for toppings
- ½ teaspoon of vanilla extract

Directions

- Take a bowl and add cream cheese. Use electric hand mixture and mix the cream cheese for about 2 minutes until thick peak formed
- Take another bowl add heavy whipping cream, sweetener, vanilla extract and mix them for about 2 minutes until thick fluffy mixture is formed
- Take a bowl add all the ingredients and top them with strawberries and blueberries at the top
- Store them in the refrigerator for about 30 minutes
- Serve them chilled

Recipe No 5

Keto Chocolate Chip Cookies

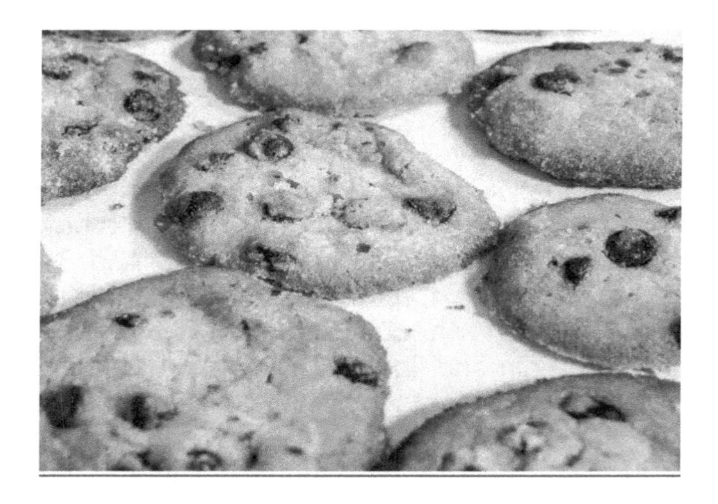

Preparing Time: 20 minutes,
Cooking Time: 20 minutes
Serving: 3 people

Ingredients

- 3 ounces of salted butter
- 3 cups of erythritol
- 1 teaspoon of vanilla extract
- 1 golden egg
- 2 cups of almond flour
- ½ teaspoon of baking powder
- ¼ teaspoon of salt
- 2 cups of sugar-free chocolate chip

Directions

- Preheat the air fryer oven at 180 degrees
- Take a nonstick pan, add butter, let it melt on medium heat for 4 minutes then pour the butter in a bowl, add erythritol and beat them until well combined. Then add egg, and vanilla extract. Beat them on low flame until well combined for about 15 minutes
- Slowly add almond flour, baking powder and some salt. Stir all the ingredients together until well combined
- Press the dough in the bowl by using your hands. Then put the dough on the tray and knead them by adding chocolate chip
- Scoop the dough on the air fryer basket lined with parchment paper and make 13 cookies and bake them for about 15 minutes until they are turned into crispy and golden brown
- After 7 minutes of baking press the cookies by using spatula and cook them for the rest of the time
- Then serve it at room temperature and you can also store them in the container for later use

Recipe No 6

Keto Mug Cake

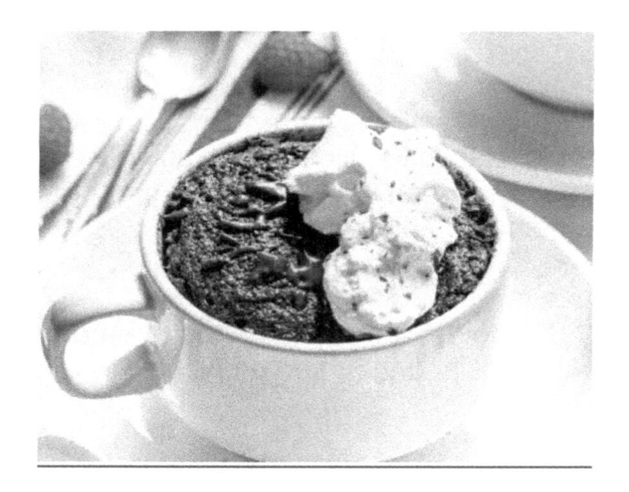

Preparing Time: 2 minutes,
Cooking Time: 1 minute
Serving: 1 people

Ingredients

- 3 tablespoon of almond flour
- 2 tablespoons of cocoa powder
- 1 teaspoon of sugar
- ½ teaspoon of baking powder
- 1 tablespoon of mayonnaise
- 1 large egg yolk
- 2 tablespoons of water

Directions

- After measuring all the ingredients in a mug, add all the dry ingredients in it. Mix them by using wooden spoon
- Then add mayonnaise, water and egg yolk
- Stir them to combine well
- Let them sit aside for 2 minutes
- Microwave it for 30 seconds
- After 30 seconds remove from the oven and store them in refrigerator and then serve chilled

Recipe No 7

Keto Low Carb Blueberry Crisps

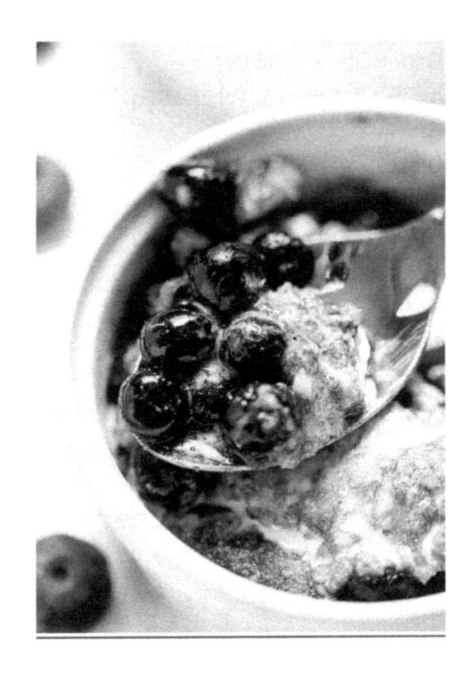

Preparing Time: 10 minutes,
Cooking Time: 15minute
Serving: 1 people

Ingredients

- 1 cup of frozen blueberries
- ½ cup of pecan halves
- 3 tablespoons of almond flour
- 1 tablespoon of butter
- 3 tablespoons of granulated sweetener
- 1 tablespoon of flaxseeds
- ½ teaspoon of cinnamon powder
- ½ teaspoon of vanilla extract
- Some kosher salt to taste
- 2 tablespoons of heavy whipping cream

Directions

- Preet heat the oven at 180 F
- Take a ramekin cup, add blueberries and sweetener. Stir them to combine
- Take a food processor and add almond flour, pecans, butter, sweetener, flax seed, cinnamon powder, kosher salt and vanilla extract. Blend them until well combined
- Now spread this mixture on the top of the blueberries mixture. And then bake them for about 15 minutes until the it turns golden brown and crispy
- Serve them

Recipe No 8

Sugar Free Chocolate Bark With Bacon And Almonds

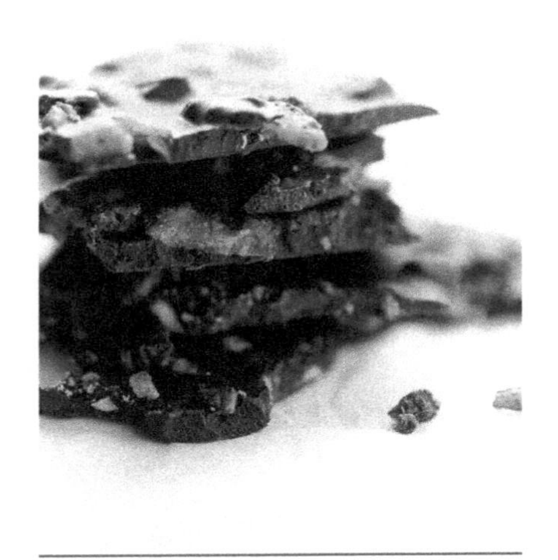

Preparing Time: 5 minutes,
Cooking Time: 25 minute's
Serving: 3 people

Ingredients

- 20 ounces bag of chocolate chips
- 1 cup of chopped almonds
- 3 slices of bacon cooked and crumbled

Directions

- Take a microwave safe bowl, microwave the chocolate chips for 2 minutes while continuously stirring
- Now add the chopped almonds in the melted chocolate and then stir them
- Now pour the melted chocolate in the tin layer pan lined with the parchment paper. And then sprinkle the crumbled bacon on the top of the chocolate layer
- Now refrigerate the chocolate later for about 20 minutes
- Then peel the parchment paper then cut then into pieces
- Serve them and enjoy

Recipe No 9

Keto Brown Butter Pralines

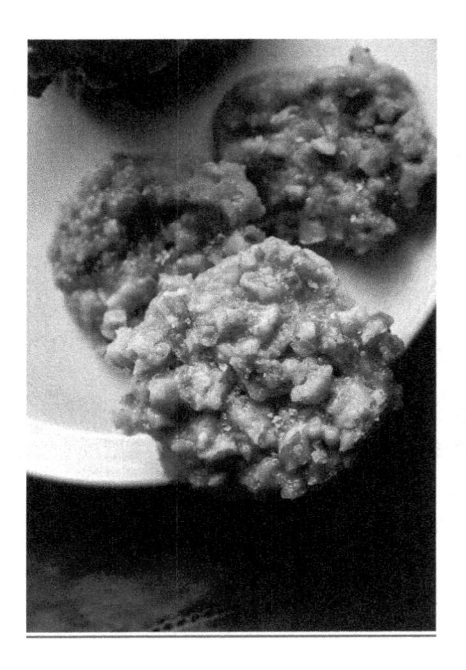

Preparing Time: 2 minutes,
Cooking Time: 60 minute's
Serving: 3 people

Ingredients

- 3 sticks of unsalted butter
- 2 cups of heavy whipping cream
- 2 cups of granular sweetener
- ½ teaspoon of xanthan gum
- 2 cups of pecan
- Some kosher salt to taste

Directions

- Prepare a baking sheet with a lined parchment sheet
- Take a nonstick pan, add butter, stir them on a low flame. Then add xanthan gums, heavy cream, and sweetener. Stir them continuously until they are well combined
- Now add nuts in the same pan and stir them continuously until they are mixed together
- Now refrigerate this mixture occasionally stirring for 1 hour.
- Now scoop this thick and sticky mixture into the cookies and then sprinkle with some maldon salt.
- Let these cookies refrigerate for 1 hour.
- You can store this in the container

Recipe No 10

The Best Keto CheeseCake

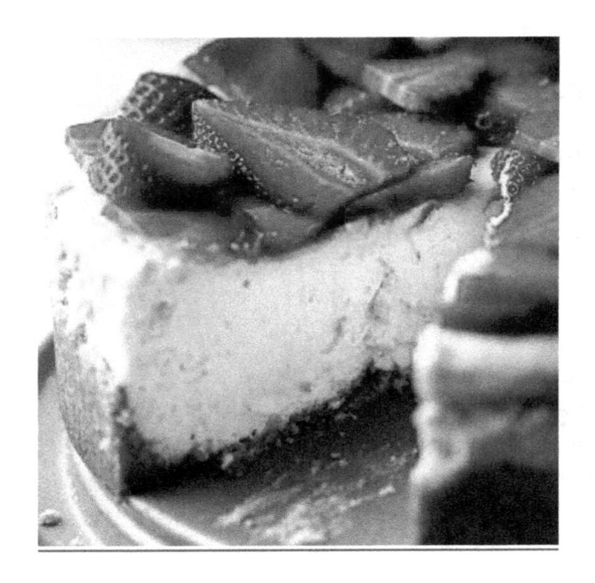

Preparing Time: 20 minutes,
Cooking Time: 50 minute's
Serving: 12 people

Ingredients

For The Crust

- 2 cups of almond flour
- 3 tablespoons of powdered sweetener
- 1 teaspoon of ground cinnamon
- 7 tablespoons of melted butter

For The Filling

- 3 cups of cream cheese
- 2 cups of powdered sweetener
- 5 golden eggs
- 8 ounces of sour cream cheese
- 1 tablespoon of vanilla extract

Directions

- Preheat the oven at 180 F
- Now adjust the rack in the middle of the oven
- Take a bowl and add the dry ingredients in the butter. Pour this dry ingredients crust in the pan and then press the crust by using your fingers then refrigerate the crust for up-to 20 minutes
- Now take a bowl, add cream cheese and beat them by using an electric hand mixer until they become fluffy. The add the sweetener and mix then again beat them by using an electric hand mixer
- Add the eggs and beat them in the cream cheese mixer. Then add vanilla extract and sour cream.
- Mix them until smooth creamy mixture is formed
- Now pour the cream cheese mixture on the top of the crust mixture. Now bake them in the preheated oven for about 50 minutes
- Turn off the oven and let the cake sit in the oven for about 30 minutes
- Now refrigerate the cake for 1 hour after 1 hour remove the cake and top with your favorite toppings

- Serve them and enjoy

Recipe No 11

Keto Chicken And Broccoli Casserole

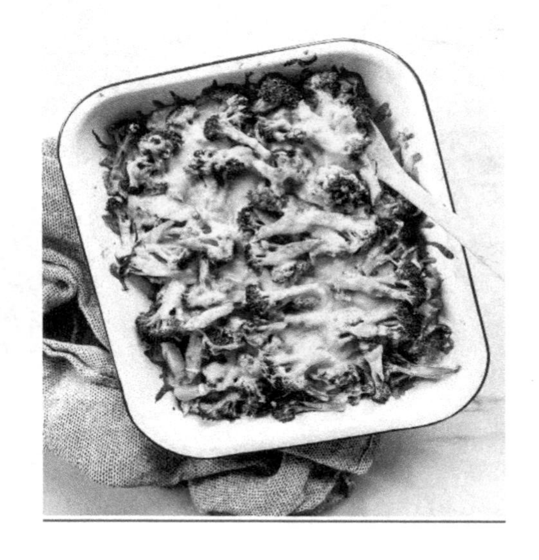

Preparing Time: 20 minutes,
Cooking Time: 30 minute's
Serving: 12 people

Ingredients

- 2 tablespoons of extra virgin olive oil
- 2 ½ cups of cooked chicken, cut into bite-sized pieces
- 2 cups of chopped and cooked broccoli
- ¼ cup of sliced almonds
- 4 tablespoons of butter
- 1 cup of heavy cream
- 8 ounces package of cream cheese cut into 1-inches cube
- 4 ounces of grated cheddar cheese
- Some kosher salt to taste
- Some ground black pepper to taste
- ¾ cups of pork rind

Directions

- Preheat the oven at 350 degrees F
- Pour olive oil in the baking dish and spread all over the bottom and sides. Place the chicken in a single layer in the bottom of the dish. Distribute the cooked broccoli evenly over the chicken and sprinkle with almonds
- Melt the butter in a saucepan over medium heat. Add cream, cook and stir them for 2-3 minutes Stir in the cream cheese and stir until melted for 2-3 minutes. Season them with salt and pepper. Pour sauce over chicken, broccoli and almonds. Top them with the crushed pork rinds
- Bake in the preheat oven until sauce is bubbly for 25 to 30 minutes

Recipe No 12

Keto BBQ Ribs

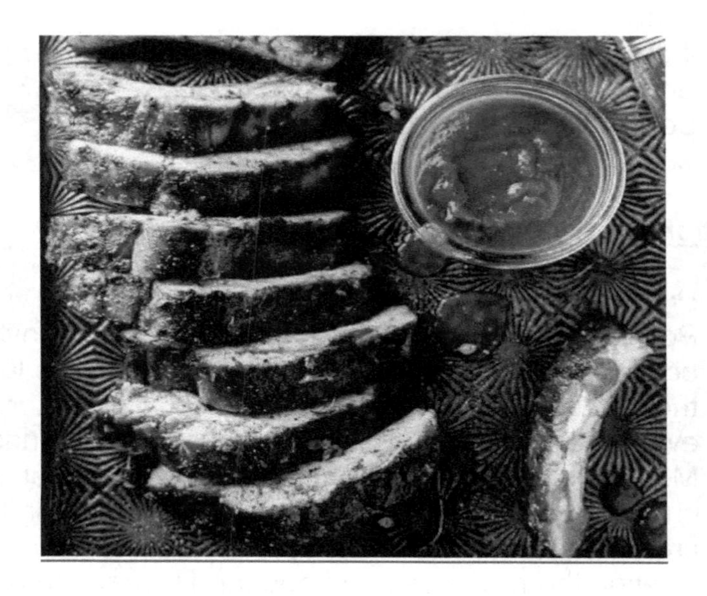

Preparing Time: 20 minutes,
Cooking Time: 4 hrs and 10 minute's
Serving: 12 people

Ingredients

- 2 tablespoons of kosher salt
- 1 tablespoon of smoked paprika
- ½ teaspoon of onion powder
- ½ teaspoon of garlic powder
- ½ teaspoon of black pepper
- 1 sheet of heavy-duty aluminum foil
- 6 pounds of pork ribs
- 2 cups of wood chips
- 1 cup of water
- 1 teaspoon of vegetable oil
- 1 keto BBQ sauce

Directions

- Take a small bowl and add salt, paprika, onion powder, garlic powder, ginger powder and black pepper. Stir them to combine all the ingredients
- Place one layer of aluminum foil on a baking sheet leaving about 2 inch overhang on all sides
- Pat the ribs dry using a paper towel and rub spice mixture into both side's of the ribs. Place the rib racks meat side up on a prepared baking sheet. Cover with more aluminum foil and lightly crimp the edges. Refrigerate then for 8-24 hours
- Preheat the oven at 225 degrees F
- Place the covered baking sheet on the centre rack of the oven and bake them for 4 hours. Remove then from the oven and rest ribs for 10 minutes
- Place the wood chips in a bowl and cover with water. Preheat an outdoor grill on medium heat
- Drain the wood chips and place in an aluminum foil packet. Pok several holes in the packet. Place the wood chip packet on the hottest part of the grill and close the lid
- When the chips are smoking oil the grate between the

ribs rack will go. Remove the ribs from the foil and place the rib racks on the oiled grate. Brush them with the BBQ sauce. Close the lid and grill them for 5-10 minutes monitoring closely for flare ups. Turn ribs and baste the other side with remaining BBQ sauce

- Close the lid and grill, again monitoring for flare ups for an additional 5-10 minutes. Keep turning and blasting until the ribs reach your desired color. Slice the ribs into portions and serve them with an additional BBQ sauce
- Enjoy

Recipe No 13

Keto Shrimps Scampi

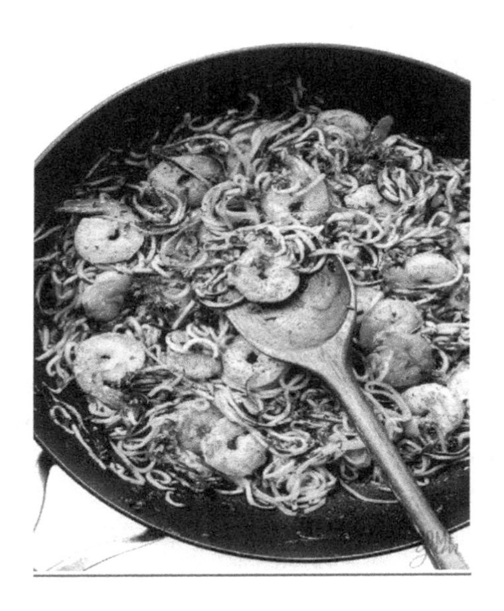

Preparing Time: 10 minutes,
Cooking Time: 25 minute's
Serving: 3 people

Ingredients

- 8 ounces package of shirataki noodles, drained and rinsed
- 1 tablespoon of olive oil
- 1 tablespoon of minced shallot
- 2 cloves of garlic minced
- ¼ teaspoon of red pepper flakes
- 12 ounces of raw shrimps peeled, and deveined
- ¼ tablespoon of salt
- ⅛ teaspoon of ground black pepper
- 3 tablespoons of white wine
- 2 tablespoon of butter
- 1 tablespoon of freshly chopped parsley

Directions

- Cover shirataki noodles with water and bring to a boil. Boil them for 5 minutes, Drain
- Return the drained noodles to a saucepan and cook over medium heat to remove any excess moisture for 5-6 minutes. Remove them from the heat and set aside
- Drizzle the olive oil into a large skillet over medium heat. Add the shallots and stir them until translucent for 2-3 minutes. Take care not to burn
- Add garlic and pepper flakes, stir them for 1 minute. Add shrimp and cook for 2-3 minutes per side, raking care not to overcook. Season them with salt and black pepper
- Transfer the shrimps to a bowl, reserving pan dipping in the skillet. Whisk white wine and lemon juice in the skillet. Add butter and cook until fully incorporated and sauce began to thick slightly foe 2-3 minutes
- Return shrimp to the skillet. Add noodles. Sprinkle with parsley and toss to combine
- Enjoy

Recipe No 14

Low Carbs Bacon Cheese Casserole

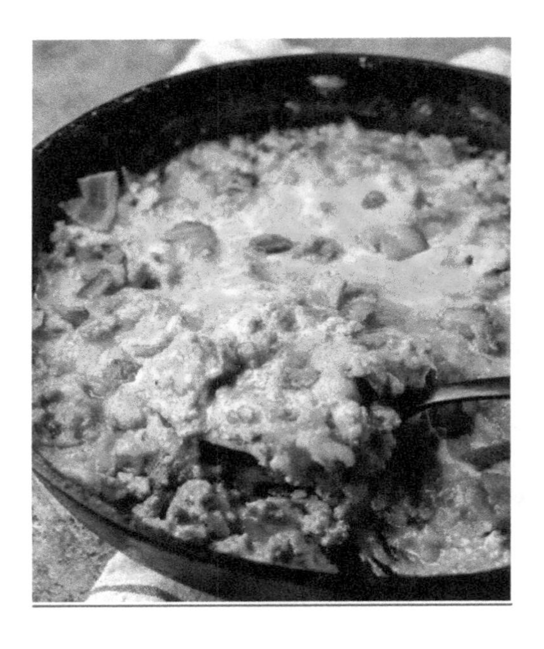

Preparing Time: 15 minutes,
Cooking Time: 35 minute's
Serving: 12 people

Ingredients

- 2 pounds of ground beef
- 2 cloves of garlic minced
- ½ teaspoon of onion powder
- 1 pound of bacon cooked, cut into pieces
- 8 large golden eggs
- 1 cup of heavy whipping cream
- ½ teaspoons of Salt
- ½ teaspoon of ground black pepper
- 12 ounces package of shredded cheddar cheese, divided

Directions

- Preheat the oven at 375 degrees F
- Heat the skillet over medium-high heat. Cook and stir beef with garlic and onion powder until browned and crumbly for 7 minutes. Drain and discardtge grease
- Spread the beef onto the bottom of the casserole pan. Stir in the bacon pieces
- Whisk eggs, heavy cream, salt and pepper in a medium bowl until well combined. Stir in 8 ounces of cheddar cheese
- Bake in the preheated oven until golden brown on top for 30 to 35 minutes
- Enjoy

Recipe No 15

Keto Chicken Breast Pot Pie With Cauliflower Crust

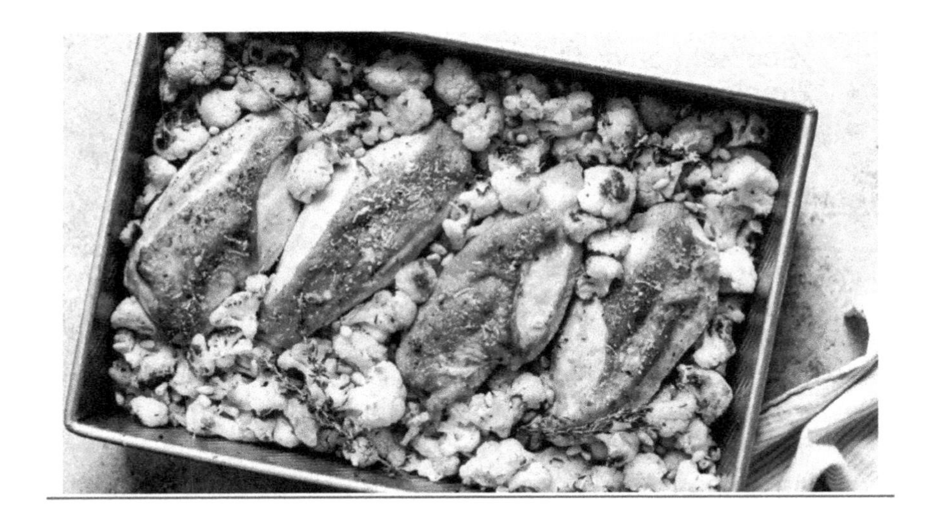

Preparing Time: 30 minutes,
Cooking Time: 60 minute's
Serving: 2 people

Ingredients

- 21 ounces of cauliflower, cut into florets with 1-inch of stalk
- ½ cup of shredded cheddar cheese
- ½ teaspoon of salt
- ½ teaspoon ground black pepper, divided
- 1 ½ ounces bacon
- ⅓ cup of diced onion
- ⅓ cup of diced carrots
- ⅓ cup of chopped celery
- 7 ½ ounces of chicken breasts
- ⅓ cup of frozen peas
- 2 tablespoons of cremini mushrooms sliced
- ½ cup of heavy whipping cream
- 2 tablespoons of cornstarch
- 1 ½ tablespoons of water

Directions

- Preheat the oven at 375 degrees
- Line the baking tray with parchment paper
- Take a food processor add the cauliflower florets and process them until it resembles rice. Transfer them to the microwave tray and bake them for about 5 minutes
- Set them aside and let them cool
- Bake them in the preheated oven for about 8 minutes. Stir them continuously whole baking for additional 7 minutes
- Remove the cauliflower from the oven and set the aside and let it cool
- Increase the oven to 400 degrees F
- Put cooled cauliflower rice in a bowl. Then add cheddar cheese, salt, black pepper, and eggs then mix them together until well combined. Press this cauliflower rice into the baking pan and spread them and make a crust
- Bake in the preheated oven for about 25 minute
- Meanwhile, heat an iron skillet over medium heat and cook the bacon until crispy and the fat has tendered.

Then add carrots, celery and onion until softened for 5 minutes. Add the chicken breasts and let them cook for about 7 minutes

- Pour the chicken broth over the chicken mixture. Season with salt and pepper. Reduce the heat and simmer at low boil until sauce has reduced to one fourth, about 5 minutes
- Mix together water and cornstarch in a bowl and create a pastry. Add them slowly in the chicken mixture while continuously stirring, until the sauce is thickened. Pour chicken mixture into the preheated cauliflower crust. Top with the remaining ½ cup of cheddar cheese

Recipe No 16

Keto Spinach Artichok

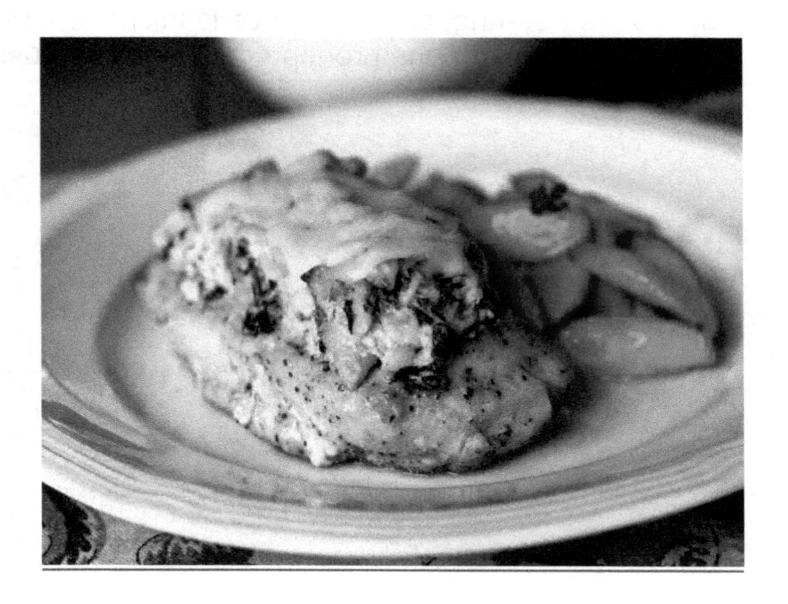

Preparing Time: 20 minutes,
Cooking Time: 30 minute's
Serving: 4 people

Ingredients

- 10 ounces package of frozen spinach
- 4 ounces package of cream cheese softened
- 14 ounces can of quartered artichoke hearts, drained and chopped
- ¼ cup of shredded Parmesan cheese
- ¼ cup of mayonnaise
- ½ teaspoon of garlic powder
- Some kosher salt to taste
- 8 ounces of boneless chicken breasts
- Pinch of salt to taste
- Some ground black pepper to taste
- 1 teaspoon of olive oil
- ½ cup of shredded mozzarella cheese

Directions

- Microwave the spinach in a bowl until warmed through for 2 to 3 minutes. Let them squeeze slightly to remove the excess moisture
- Return the spinach to the bowl. Mix in then cream cheese, artichoke hearts, Parmesan cheese, mayonnaise, garlic powder and salt. Set then aside
- Pound the chicken breasts to an even thickness, not more than 1 inch thick. Season them with salt and pepper on both sides
- Preheat the oven at 375 degrees F
- Heat the oil in a skillet over medium-high heat. Brown the chicken breast in the hot oil for 2 to 3 minutes. Working in batches if necessary. Place the chicken breasts in a large baking dish. Spread the spinach artichoke mixture on top of each breast
- Bake in the preheat oven until the chicken is no longer pink in the centre and juices run clear, for 20 to 22 minutes. Top the breast with mozzarella cheese and continue baking until the cheese has melted for more 1 or 2 minutes
- Serve them and enjoy

Recipe No 17

Keto Lemon Garlic Chicken Thighs In The Air Fryer

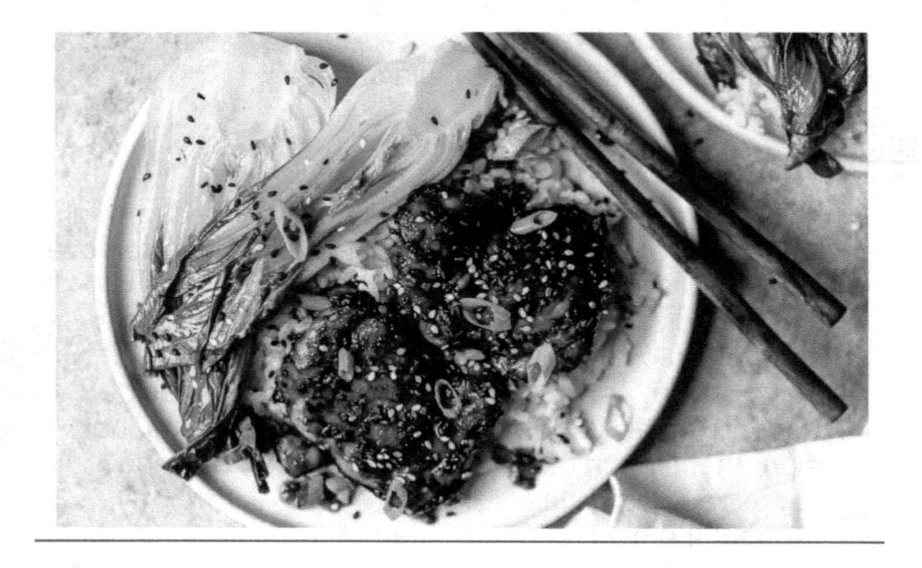

Preparing Time: 20 minutes,
Cooking Time: 30 minute's
Serving: 4 people

Ingredients

- ¼ cup of lemon juice
- 2 tablespoons of olive oil
- 1 tablespoon of Dijon mustard
- 2 cloves of minced garlic
- ¼ teaspoon of salt
- ⅛ teaspoon of ground black pepper
- 4 inches of boneless chicken thighs (2)
- 4 wedge (blank) lemon wedges

Directions

- Take a bowl add lemon juice, olive oil, Dijon mustard, salt and black pepper to taste. Stir all the ingredients together until well combined
- Place the chicken thighs in a resealable plastic bag. Pour the marinade over the chicken and seal the bag making sure to cover all the parts of the chicken
- Refrigerate them for at least 2 hours
- Preheat an air fryer to at least 375 F
- Remove the chicken from the marinade and pat dry with a paper towel. Place these chicken pieces in an air fryer basket, cooking in batches if necessary
- Fry the chicken until it doesn't remains pink at the bone and juices run clear, 22 to 24 minutes. Squeeze the lemon wedges ovee each piece before serving. Top them with your favorite veggies and enjoy

Recipe No 18

Keto Meatballs

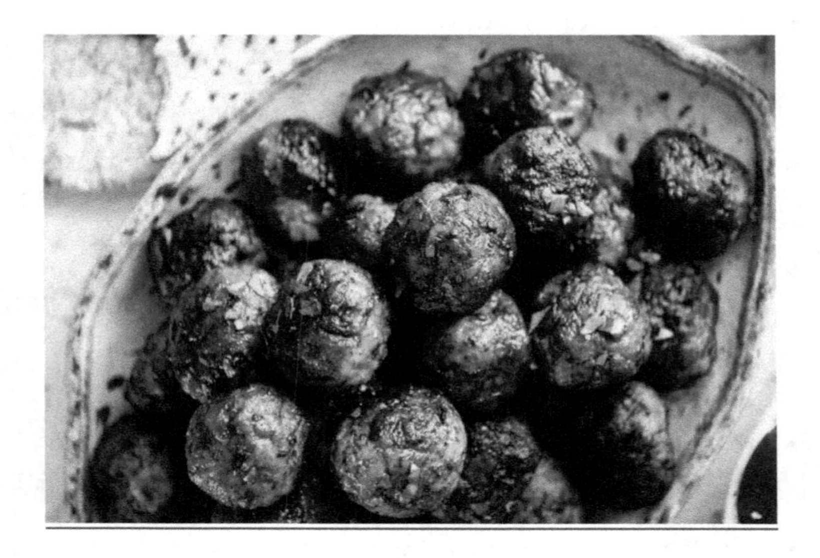

Preparing Time: 30 minutes,
Cooking Time: 15 minute's
Serving: 6 people

Ingredients

- 1 pound of ground chicken
- ⅓ cup of blanched almonds flour
- ½ teaspoon of salt
- ½ teaspoon of garlic powder
- ½ teaspoon of onion powder
- 1 egg lightly beaten
- 6 ounces of ham steak, cubed into 20 even pieces
- 1 tablespoon of olive oil
- 1 tablespoon of butter
- ¾ cup of chicken broth
- 1 tablespoon of Dijon mustard
- ½ cup of heavy whipping cream
- ½ cup of shredded swiss cheese
- Pinch of cracked black pepper to taste
- 2 tablespoons of finely chopped parsley
- 1 egg

Directions

- Take a bowl combine, chicken, almond flour, salt, pepper, egg, garlic powder and onion powder in the bowl. Mix then by using your hands
- Take an ice-cream scoop and make the 20 meatballs by using your hands
- Heat the olive oil in the skillet then add the meatballs in the skillet and cook them until they turned into golden brown
- Transfer the meatballs in a clean plate
- Now take another skillet and add butter add the chicken broth and Dijon mustard and bring them to simmer for 3 to 4 minutes
- Now pour this mixture into the heavy cream and whisk them until smooth creamy mixture formed. Season them with cracked black pepper and parsley. Serve them immediately. Sauce will further thicken upon cooling

- Serve them and enjoy

Recipe No 19

Keto Friendly Soup

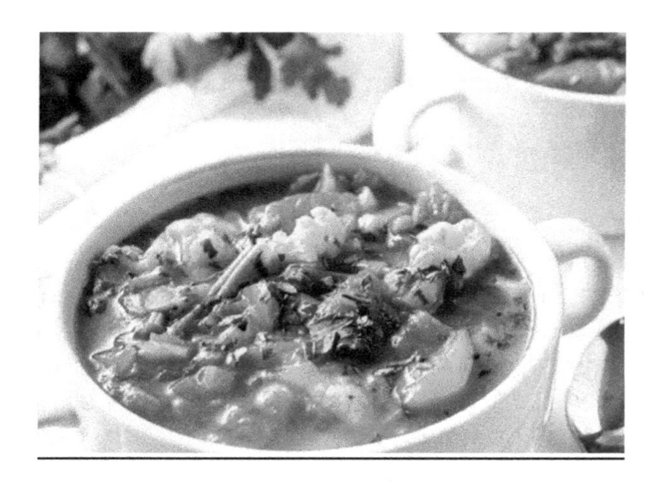

Preparing Time: 30 minutes,
Cooking Time: 15 minute's
Serving: 6 people

Ingredients

- 2 tablespoons of extra virgin olive oil
- 1 onion in diced form
- 3 red bell peppers (in diced form)
- 4 cloves of minced garlic
- 1 head of cauliflower cut into 1-inch florets
- 2 cups of green beans
- Some kosher salt to taste
- Some ground black pepper to taste
- 2 bay leaves (dried)
- 1 tablespoon of Italian seasoning
- 2 can's of diced tomatoes
- 8 cups of chicken broth

Directions

- Take a Dutch oven and turn on the flame. Add the olive oil.
- Add the onions and bell peppers. Saute them for 7 minutes until they are turned into golden brown
- Then add the minced garlic and saute them for minute
- Then add all the veggies and chicken broth. Then adjust the salt and black pepper to taste. Stir them continuously and then add bay leaves
- Cook them and let them simmer for about 20 minutes until the veggies are soft and tendered

Recipe No 20

Keto Friendly Barbecued Banana Prawns

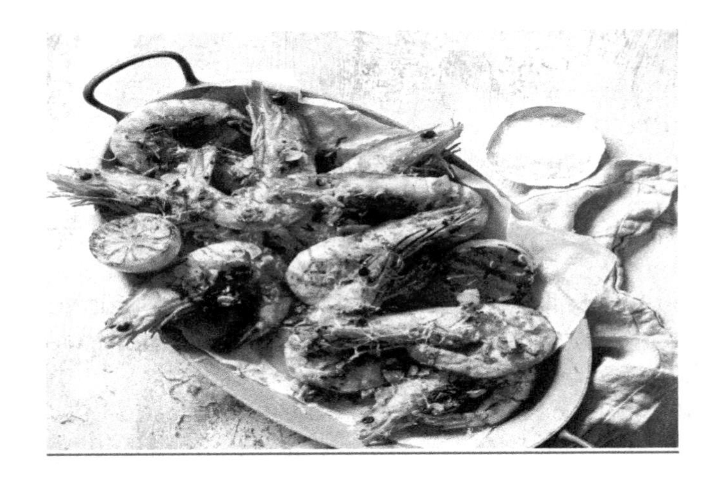

Preparing Time: 10 minutes,
Cooking Time: 10 minute's
Serving: 4 people

Ingredients

- 16 prawns (In King Size)
- 2 tablespoons of olive oil
- 200 grams of western star spreadable original
- 2 cloves of garlic thinly sliced
- 1 long red chilli, chopped
- 2 tablespoons of flat leaf parsley, chopped
- 2 tablespoons of lemon juice
- Some kosher salt to taste
- Some ground black pepper to taste

Directions

- Melt the western star spreadable in a nonstick pan on medium flame
- Once it is melted add garlic and chilli and cook them for about 1 minute
- After that remove from the flame and add chopped parsley, lemon zest and lemon juice. Stir them to combine all the ingredients until well combined
- Then sprinkle some salt and black pepper to taste. Again stir them to mix it
- Now preheat the grill and take a bowl add prawns and add olive oil toss them to coat well then putting the grill to cook and cut the lemons in half and place on the grill to caramelized
- After that place the prawns in a plate and drizzle some garlic sauce over them
- Serve them with the caramelized lemon wedges and salad
- Enjoy

Recipe No 21

Keto Friendly Creamy Avocado Zoodles

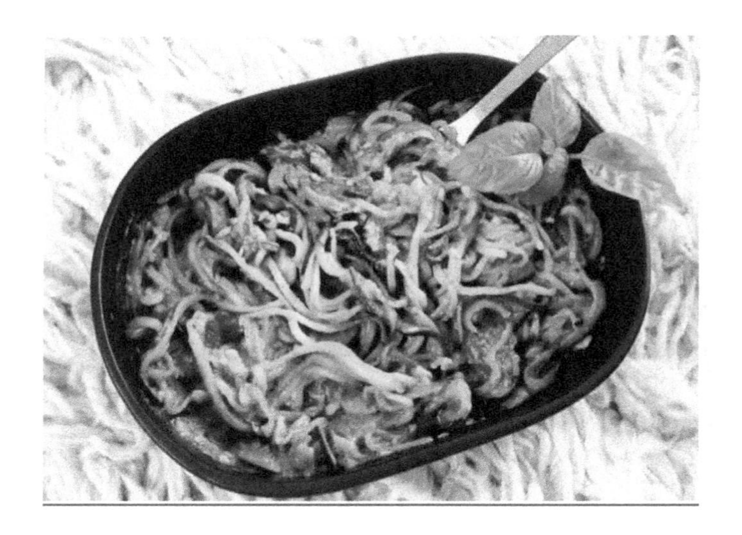

Preparing Time: 10 minutes,
Cooking Time: 10 minute's
Serving: 4 people

Ingredients

- 6 large sized zucchini
- 1 large sized avocado
- 2 cloves of minced garlic
- 1 cup of fresh basil leaves
- 1 tablespoon of lemon juice
- 1 teaspoon of extra virgin olive oil
- 1 teaspoon of nutritional yeast
- Some splash of rice bran oil
- Some kosher salt to taste
- Some ground black pepper to taste

Directions

- Take a bowl add zucchini remove it's ends and then wash them
- Take another bowl and hold a spiralizer. Spiralizer all the zucchini
- Take a non stick pan add olive oil and put the zucchini and cook the zucchini in the pan until they are softened
- Then put a splash of rice bran oil on it
- Then take a small bowl add the avocado mashed them by using fork
- Mix the olive oil, nutritional yeast and freshly chopped basil
- Now in a pan add the minced garl8c cool them. Add them in the mashed avocado then add some lemon juice. Stir them to combine and make a creamy mixture
- Now serve the spiralized zucchini in a dish and drizzle the avocados sauce on them sandstorm them
- Enjoy

Recipe No 22

Baked Sausage Ratatouille

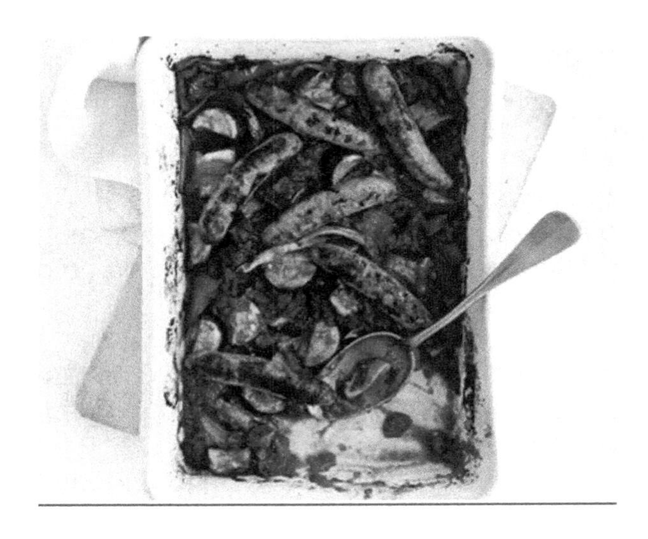

Preparing Time: 10 minutes,
Cooking Time: 40 inute's
Serving: 4 people

Ingredients

- 1 large onion cut in wedges form
- 4 courgette cut in the bite sized pieces
- 2 red small sized bell peppers cut in bite-sized pieces
- 2 tablespoons of extra virgin olive oil
- 8 sausages
- 3 cloves of garlic crushed
- 3 can's of tomatoes chopped
- Some kosher salt to taste
- Some ground black pepper to taste

Directions

- Heat the oven at 375 degrees F
- Take an oven safe baking dish add the onions, courgettes, bell peppers, then drizzle some olive oil and then season them
- Bake them for about 20 minutes
- Till then take a nonstick pan add olive oil, and cook the sausages for about 5 minutes until they are tendered or golden brown
- Then add crushed garlic cloves and chopped tomatoes in the sausages and stir them for about 4 minutes until they are tendered or mixed together
- Now remove the baking tray and set aside then drizzle the sausages on the top of the baked ingredients and then return the baking tray back to the oven and then bake them for additional 20 minutes
- After that remove them and serve
- Enjoy

Recipe N0 23

Keto Friendly Salmon With Tahini Dressing

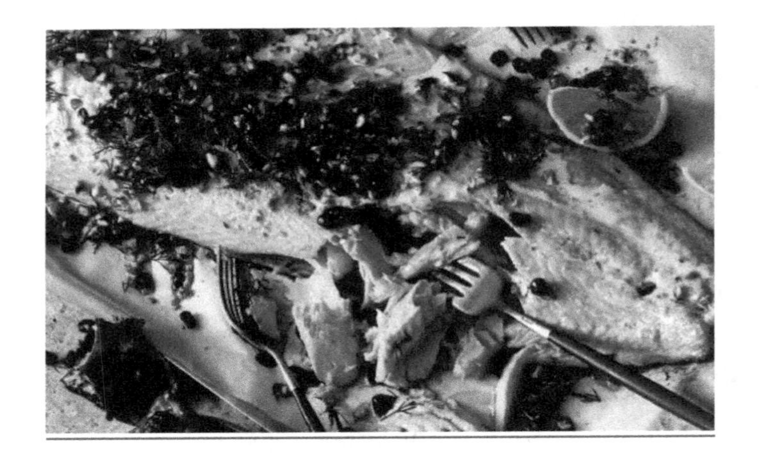

Preparing Time: 15 minutes,
Cooking Time: 20 minutes
Serving: 6 people

Ingredients

- 1 large size salmon
- 1 tablespoon of olive oil
- Small bunch of dill finely chopped
- 3 tablespoons of pistachios finely chopped
- 3 tablespoons of pomegranate seeds
- 2 tablespoon of lemon juice
- 2 tablespoons of walnut oil
- Some kosher salt to taste
- Some ground black pepper to taste

Ingredients For Tahini Dressing

- 3 tablespoons of tahini
- 1 clove of garlic minced
- 1 tablespoon of lemon juice
- ½ teaspoon of cumin powder
- ⅓ cup of water
- Some kosher salt to taste
- Some ground black pepper to taste

Directions

- Preheat an oven at 400 degrees F
- Then line the large baking tray in the oven with parchment paper
- Put the salmon and drizzle some olive oil and spread the oil all over the salmon. Then bake them for 20 minutes until it is cooked. Then remove them and place them in a plate and let them rest for about 5 minutes
- Take a bowl and add all the tahini dressing ingredients. Stir them t9 combine well until it is reached to the desired consistency
- Take another bowl add pistachios, pomegranate seeds and dill. Then spread them on the fish then drizzle the lemon juice, dill and tahini dressing on the fish. Then sprinkle some ground black pepper and salt
- Serve them and enjoy

Recipe No 24

Keto Friendly Tuna Poke Bowl

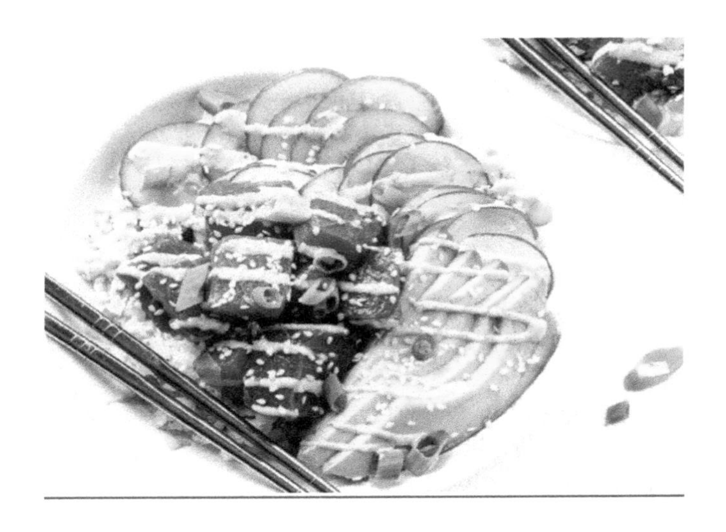

Preparing Time: 15 minutes,
Cooking Time: 5 minutes
Serving: 4 people

Ingredients

Ahi Tuna

- 5 tablespoons of coconut aminos
- 2 tablespoons of lemon juice
- 2 tablespoons of sesame oil
- 1 lbs of sushi tuna (cut into bite-sized pieces)
-

Cauliflower Rice

- 10 ounces of cauliflower rice
- 2 tablespoons of avocado oil
- Some kosher salt to taste
- Some ground black pepper to taste

Ingredients

For Pork Bowls

- 1 avocado thinly sliced
- 1 radish thinly sliced
- 1 cucumber thinly sliced
- 3 tablespoons of spicy mayonnaise
- 1 green onion finely chopped
- Some sesame seeds for garnishing

Directions

- Take a bowl add coconut aminos, lemon juice and sesame oil stir then to combine all the ingredients
- The add the tuna and toss then to coat. Refrigerate for 2 hours till then prepare the rest of the ingredients
- Take a nonstick pan and cook the cauliflower rice for about 5 minutes
- Takes bowl and add the sauce ingredients stir then to combine and pour then in the plastic seal bag with the corner snipped
- Take a bowl add the cauliflower rice, cucumber slices,

radish slices, avocado slices and Tuna.

- Squeeze the mayonnaise on the top
- Then garnish them with green onions and sesame seeds
- Serve them and enjoy

Recipe No 25

Keto Chicken Curry With Turmeric Rice

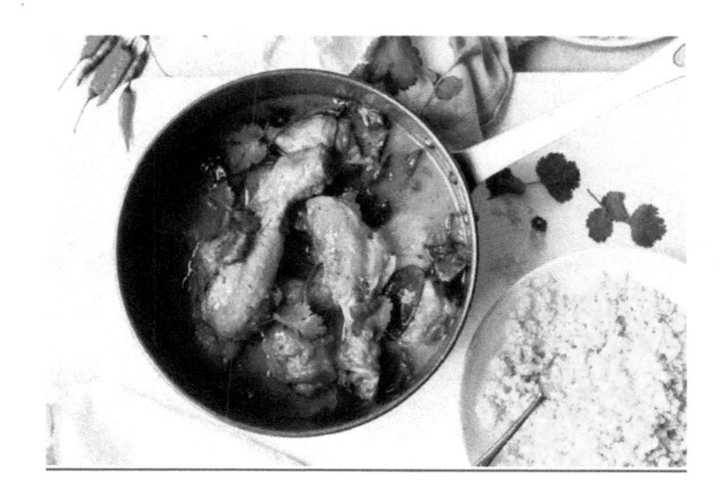

Preparing Time: 15 minutes
Cooking Time: 5 minute
Serving: 4 people

Ingredients

- 1 tablespoon of coconut oil
- 10 chicken drumsticks
- 3 tablespoons of Valcom green paste
- 2 cans of coconut cream
- 3 cups of chicken stock
- 2 kafir lime leaves
- 1 cup of baby spinach
- ½ onion thinly sliced

Cauliflower Rice

- 1 tablespoon of coconut oil
- ½ teaspoon of turmeric powder
- 500g of cauliflower rice frozen
- Some kosher salt to taste
- Some ground black pepper to taste

Directions

- Take a nonstick pan add coconut oil let it warm then add the drumsticks let it cook for about 10 minutes
- Take another bowl add curry paste and then add the chicken stir them continuously for about 5 minutes. Then add the coconut cream, chicken stock and lime leaves. Let them simmer for about 40 minutes until the chicken is tendered
- Then set them aside
- Take another skillet and add the coconut oil and add the turmeric powder. Then add the cauliflower rice and water. Let them cook for about 7 minutes. Sprinkle some salt and black pepper
- Then serve the curry with the cauliflower rice.
- Serve them and Enjoy

Recipe No 26

Baked Salmon Fillet With Raw Broccoli Salad

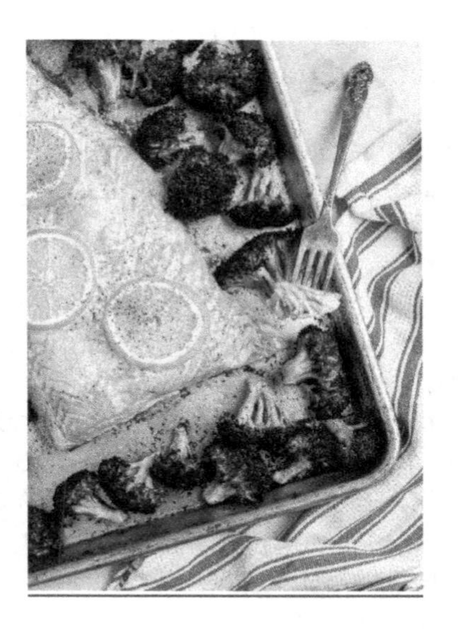

Preparing Time: 5 minutes,
Cooking Time: 20 minutes
Serving: 4 people

Ingredients

- 1 pound of salmon
- 2 broccoli crowns cut into florets
- 4 tablespoons of melted butter
- 3 tablespoons of butter
- Some sliced lemon wedges
- Some kosher salt to taste
- Some ground black pepper to taste

Directions

- Take a baking sheet pan, add the cauliflower florets on the sides of the pan then drizzle some olive oil. Toss them to coat
- Add the salmon in the centre of the pan brush the melted butter and top them with the lemon slices. Sprinkle some salt and black pepper to taste
- Now add the baking pan in the oven and cook them for about 20 minutes in the oven and then serve them with sauce and enjoy

Recipe No 27

Keto Friendly Lamb Tagine

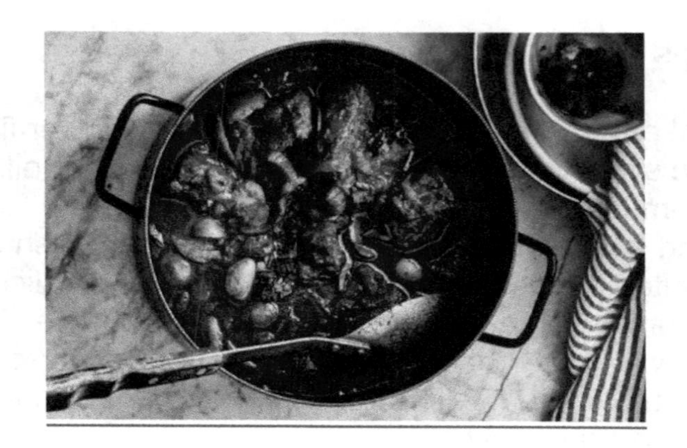

Preparing Time: 20 minutes,
Cooking Time: 2 hours
Serving: 4 people

Ingredients

- 500 grams of beef onto diced form
- 1 tablespoon of extra virgin olive oil
- 2 onions peeled and finely chopped
- 2 cloves of garlic finely chopped
- 1 teaspoon of cumin powder
- 1 teaspoon of garlic powder
- 1 teaspoon of paprika powder
- 1 teaspoon of sweet pap
- 2 can's of tomatoes chopped and diced
- 1 cup of beef broth
- 2 bay leaves
- ½ cup of Kalamata olives halved pitted
- 1 red capsicum finely chopped
- Some kosher salt to taste
- Some ground black pepper to taste

Directions

- Take a nonstick pan add olive oil and then add the Onions and Garlic then saute them for 4 minutes
- Then add the spices and then add the beef. Stir them and cook them until they are tendered or turned into golden brown
- Then add the broth, tomatoes, capsicums and olives.
- Let them simmer for sometime
- Cook them for 90 minutes
- Remove the lid and allow the sauce to get it thickens
- Serve them and enjoy

Recipe No 28

Keto Friendly 20-minutes Chicken

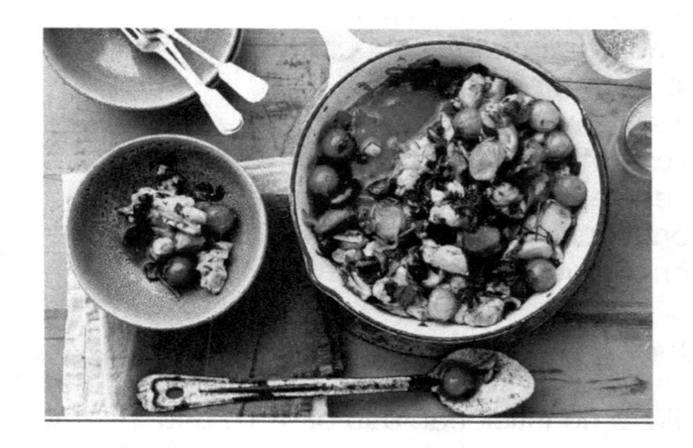

Preparing Time: 10 minutes,
Cooking Time: 20 minutes
Serving: 4 people

Ingredients

- 500 grams of chicken thighs (cut them in diced
- 2 tablespoons of extra virgin olive oil
- 1 brown onion in sliced form
- 4 cloves of garlic minced
- 2 cans of cherry tomatoes
- ¼ cup of pitted black olives
- 1 can of anchovy fillets
- 1 tablespoon of chilli flakes

Directions

- Take a large nonstick pan. Add the olive oil, then add the sliced onion and garlic. Let them saute for about 5 minutes
- Add the chicken thighs in cubed form. Let them coat in the olive oil. Cook them on high flame
- Add the chilli flakes and cook them for another 5 minutes
- Now reduce the heat on low flame and add anchovy fillets, black olives, cherry tomatoes stir them to combine and cook them for further 12 minutes
- Now Sprinkle then with salt and black pepper
- After that serve them and enjoy

Recipe No 29

Keto Friendly Zoodles And Egg Salad

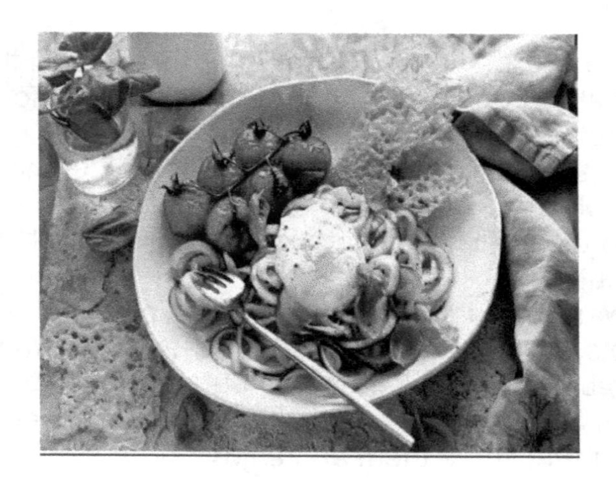

Preparing Time: 20 minutes,
Cooking Time: 30 minutes
Serving: 4 people

Ingredients

- 2 packet of sweet berry trust tomatoes
- 1 cup of grated Parmesan cheese
- 4 golden eggs
- 3 zucchini (trimmed)
- 2 tablespoons of extra virgin olive oil
- 2 cloves of garlic minced
- ½ cup of basil leaves
- Some kosher salt to taste

Directions

- Preheat the oven at 400 degrees F. Take 2 baking trays lined with parchment paper. Put the tomatoes in one baking tray, drizzle them with olive oil and in the second try put the Parmesan cheese and bake them for about 20 minutes until the tomatoes are tendered and Parmesan cheese turns into golden crispy large shards
- Take a deep pan add water and let then boil until whirlpool is formed. Now crack the egg in a small bowl and whisk them until well combined. Then slightly pour them in the whirlpool. Cook them for 3 minutes until it is totally cooked.
- with the help of slotted spoon put the egg in a plate
- With the help of spiralizer, cut the zucchini in spirals. Heat up the oil in a frying pan. Add the zucchini and garlic in the pan. Cook them for about 3 minutes. Remove them from the heat and then add basil leaves. Toss them to combine well
- Then divide the zucchini zoodles in the serving plate and then top them with the poached eggs
- Serve then at room temperature with roasted tomatoes and Parmesan crisps

Recipe No 30

Keto Ground Chicken Tacos

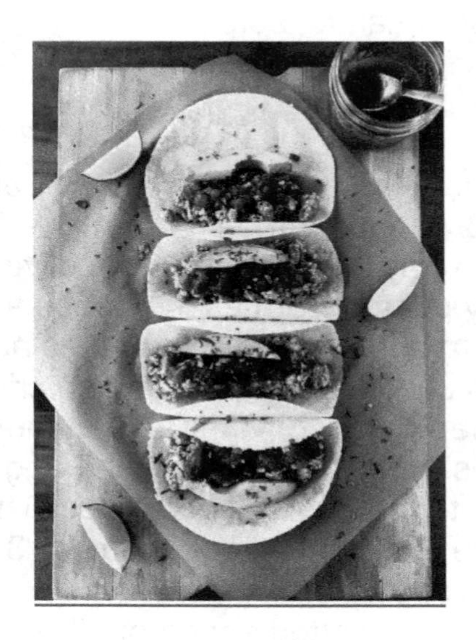

Preparing Time: 5 minutes,
Cooking Time: 15 minutes
Serving: 4 people

Ingredients

- 1 teaspoon of Cumin powder
- 1 teaspoon of Chilli powder
- 1 teaspoon of Ground coriander
- ½ teaspoon of Onion powder
- ½ teaspoon of Garlic powder
- ⅓ teaspoon of Oregano
- ⅛ teaspoon of Chipotle chilli powder
- 1 tablespoon of Avocado oil
- 1 lbs of ground chicken
- ¼ cup of chicken broth
- Some sea salt to taste
- 1 teaspoon of Lemon juice

Directions

- Take a small bowl add chilli powder, cumin powder, ground coriander, onion powder, garlic powder, orgenao and chipotle chili powder. Stir them to combine well until combined
- Take a nonstick pan add olive oil
- Add the ground chicken in a nonstick pan and break them with a spatula.
- Stir them continuously until the moisture is absorbed
- Add the spices and mix them together coat in the spices
- Add the lemon juice and chicken broth
- Toss them together until all the ingredients are well combined
- Adjust the seasonings as per your taste
- Serve them and enjoy

Recipe No 31

Keto Pizza Roll Ups

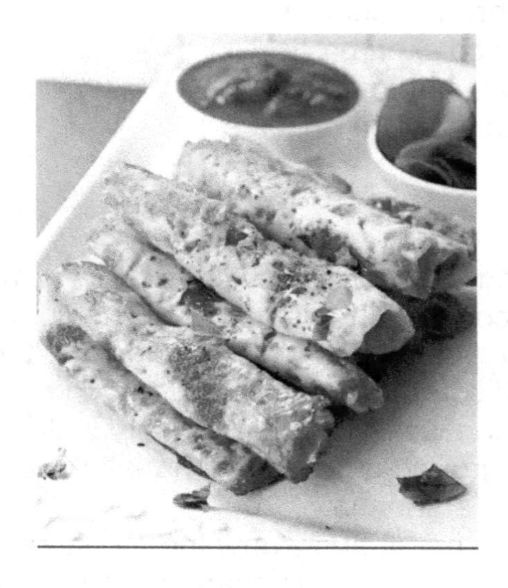

Preparing Time : 5 minutes
Cooking Time: 1 minute
Servings: 3 people

Ingredients

- Mozzarella cheese slices 12-13
- Mini pepperoni slices as many you desired
- 3 tablespoons of Italian seasoning
- 3 tablespoons of keto marina sauce

Directions

- Preheat an oven at 400 degrees F
- Then line the baking tray with a parchment paper
- Put the cheese slices in the parchment lined baking tray and let them cook for 1 minutes until their edges start to softened and turns brown
- After that remove from the oven and let the cheese slices to cool. Spread some Italian seasoning and put the pepperoni slices on the cheese slices
- Then slightly roll up and then serve them with your favorite dipping sauce and enjoy

Recipe No 32

Keto Cauliflower Mac And Cheese

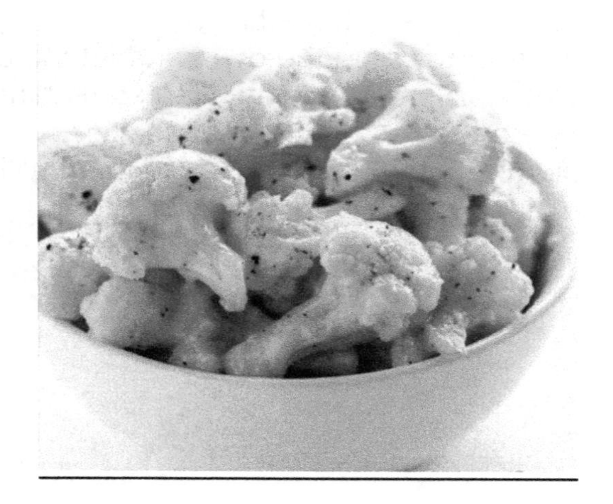

Preparing Time : 10 minutes
Cooking Time: 25 minute
Servings: 3 people

Ingredients

- 1 large head of cauliflower (Cut their florets)
- 3 tablespoons of melted butter
- Some sea salt to taste
- Some kosher salt to taste
- 1 cup of shredded cheddar cheese
- 4 tablespoons of heavy whipping cream
- 4 tablespoons of unsweetened milk

Directions

- Preheat the oven at 400 degrees F
- Line the baking tray with parchment paper
- Take a bowl add the cauliflower florets and drizzle 2 tablespoons of melted butter and sprinkle some salt and black pepper
- Gently toss them together until all the ingredients stick to the cauliflower
- Spread these cauliflower florets on the baking tray lined with parchment paper and then roast them for about 10- 15 minutes
- Take a bowl add cheddar cheese, heavy whipping cream and 1 tablespoon of melted butter. Stir them to combine and them microwave them for 30 seconds t0 melt them
- Remove the cauliflower florets from the oven, add them in a large bowl and drizzle the cheese sauce. Toss them to coat well and serve
- Enjoy

Recipe No 33

Keto Spinach Artichoke Dip

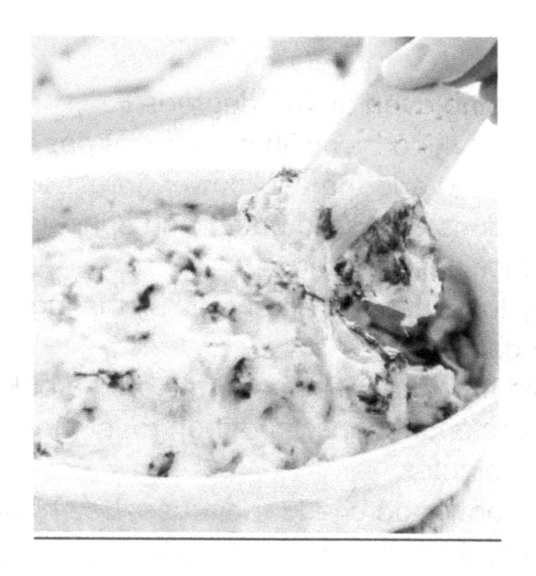

Preparing Time : 10 minutes
Cooking Time: 30 minutes
Servings: 10 people

Ingredients

- Chopped spinach 4 ounces
- Cream cheese 4 ounces
- 3 tablespoons of mayonnaise
- 2 teaspoon of sour cream
- 4 tablespoons of grated Parmesan cheese
- 1 can of artichoke hearts (water drained)
- 4 cloves of garlic minced
- Some sea salt and black pepper to taste
- 2 cups of mozzarella cheese

Directions

- Take an oil greased nonstick pan and then add the chopped spinach let them cook for about 2-3 minutes until the spinach is tendered or wilted
- Then set them aside remove the excess moisture and let then cool
- Until the spinach is cooled preheat the oven at 375 degrees F
- Take an ovenproof bowl add the cream cheese let them melt for about 30 minutes then remove them and add sour cream, mayonnaise, artichoke hearts, minced garlic, grated Parmesan cheese, some black pepper and salt and some mozzarella cheese. Stir all the ingredients together until well combined
- When the spinach is cool enough press them several times to squeeze the excess moisture
- Then transfer the spinach in an artichoke mixture.
- Then transfer the dip in a ceramic bowl and smooth the surface. Then sprinkle some shredded mozzarella cheese on the top
- Microwave them for about 30 minutes

- Then serve them and enjoy

Recipe No 34

Keto Sausage Pizza Bites

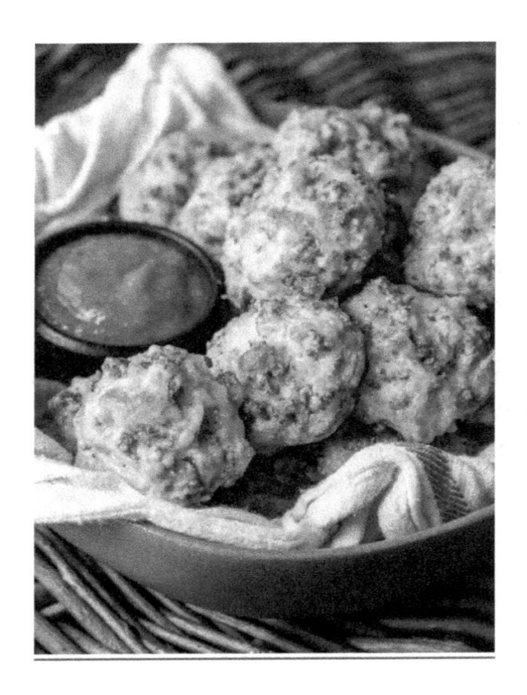

Preparing Time : 10 minutes
Cooking Time: 30 minutes
Servings: 10 people

Ingredients

- 1 pound of sausages, cooked and then drained
- 1 cup of cream cheese, softened
- 4 tablespoons of almond flour
- ½ teaspoon of baking powder
- 2 cloves of minced garlic
- 1 tablespoon of Italian seasoning
- 3 large golden eggs cracked and whisked
- 1 ¼ cup of mozzarella cheese

Directions

- Preheat the oven at 375 degrees F
- Take a bowl and add the cooked sausages and cream cheese. Stir then together until well combined
- The add the rest of the Ingredients until well combined and let them absorb the moisture
- Take a baking tray lined with parchment paper
- Take a cookie scoop and put the dough
- Place then in the oven and bake them for about 20 minutes
- Then remove the in a bowl and serve them with your favorite sauce and enjoy

Recipe No 35

Keto Stuffed Mushrooms

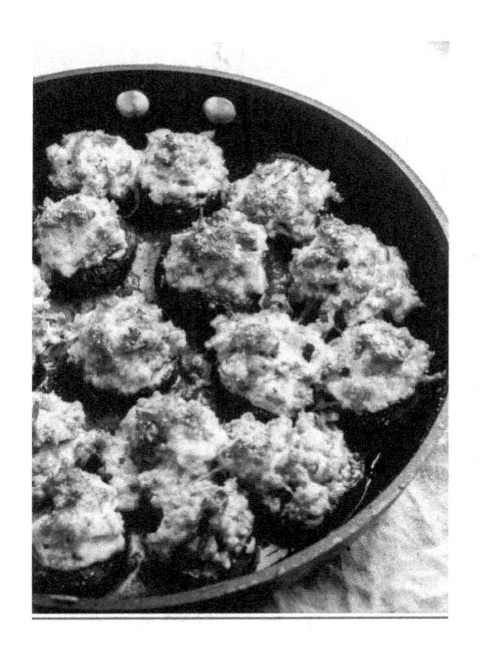

Preparing Time : 15 minutes
Cooking Time: 20 minutes
Servings: 6 people

Ingredients

- 1 lbs of Italian sausages
- 1 lbs of cremini mushrooms
- 4 ounces of cream cheese
- 4 tablespoons of mozzarella cheese
- Some sea salt to taste
- 1 teaspoon of red pepper flakes
- 4 tablespoon of grated Parmesan cheese

Directions

- Preheat the oven at 375 degrees F
- Take a nonstick pan, turn on the flame, then put the sausages and let them turn into golden brown and crispy. Remove them in a bowl
- Add the cream cheese, mozzarella cheese, stir them to combine well until all the ingredients are mixed together
- As per your taste add the seasonings
- Take an oven safe tray lined with parchment paper, put the mushroom caps and spread some sausage mixture and then sprinkle some Parmesan cheese. Then put them in the preheated oven and then bake them for about 25 minutes
- Until the cheese is turned int9 golden brown
- Serve them and enjoy

Recipe No 36

Keto Asparagus Fries

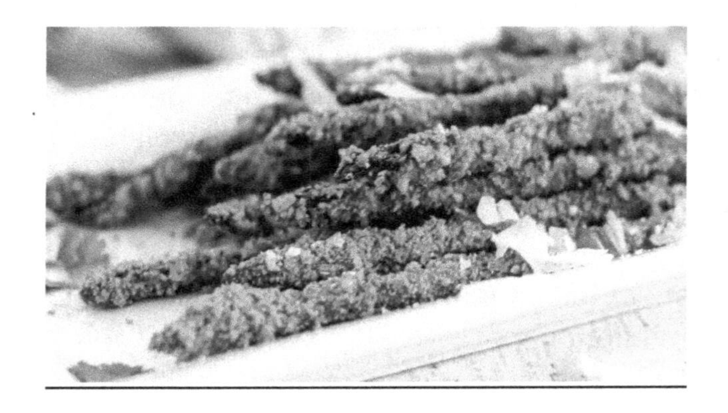

Preparing Time : 10 minutes
Cooking Time: 12 minutes
Servings: 4 people

Ingredients

- Handful of asparagus tips removed
- 3 golden eggs
- 3 tablespoons of heavy whipping cream
- 1 tablespoon of extra virgin olive oil
- 2 cups of crushed pork rinds
- Some sea salt and ground black pepper to taste
- ½ teaspoon of paprika
- 1 teaspoon of garlic powder
- ½ cup of grated Parmesan cheese
- Some shaved Parmesan cheese for garnishing
- Some freshly chopped parsley for garnish

Directions

- Preheat the air fryer basket at 400 depress F lined with parchment paper
- Take a bowl add asparagus drain them with water and cut two inches of asparagus from between the center
- Take a bowl add cream cheese, oil and golden eggs. Whisk them together until well combined
- Take a plate and add grated Parmesan cheese, crushed pork rinds, paprika powder, garlic powder, and pepper powder
- Now take an asparagus and dip them in the egg wash mixture and then coat them completely with the pork rinds mixture
- Repeat with the rest of the asparagus
- Now place the asparagus on the air fryer basket and by keeping a space between them and then bake them for about 12 minutes. After 12 minutes remove them from the air fryer basket and sprinkle the shredded Parmesan cheese and parsley.

- Serve them and enjoy

Recipe No 37

Keto Cheese Stuffed Meatballs

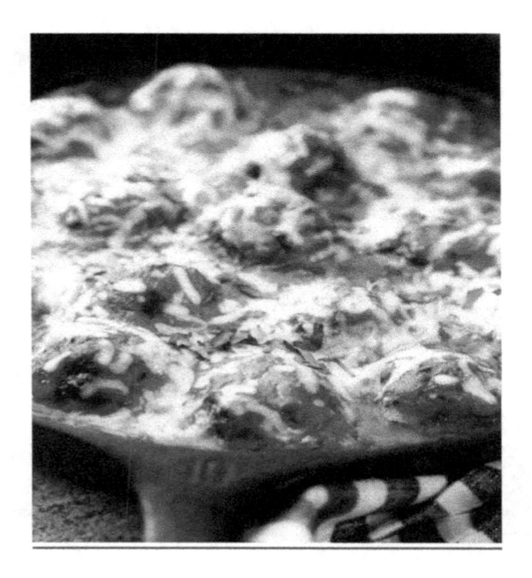

Preparing Time : 10 minutes
Cooking Time: 24 minutes
Servings: 4 people

Ingredients

- 1 pound of ground beef
- 1 pound of Italian sausages
- 1 teaspoon of oregano
- Some kosher salt to taste
- Some ground black pepper to taste
- 4 mozzarella cheese sticks cut in pieces
- 1 teaspoon of garlic powder
- 2 tablespoons of avocado oil
- 2 cans of marina sauce
- 1 cup of mozzarella cheese
- Some finely chopped parsley for garnishing

Directions

- Take a bowl add the ground beef, then add salt, pepper, Italian sausages, garlic powder, and dried oregano
- Take an ovenproof pan and add the oil
- Take another bowl add the mozzarella cheese mixture and ground beef mixture. Mix them by using your hands and then make balls by using your hands.
- Place these meatballs in the pan
- Now place this ovenproof pan in the preheated oven and cook them for about 12 minutes until they are turned into golden brown
- After 12 minutes remove the pan from the oven and pour the marina sauce and sprinkle some mozzarella cheese on the top
- Now again place the pan in the oven and bake them for about 12 minutes more
- After 12 minutes remove the pan from the oven and then serve them by garnishing some chopped parsley

Recipe No 38

Keto Bacon Wrapped Brussels Sprouts

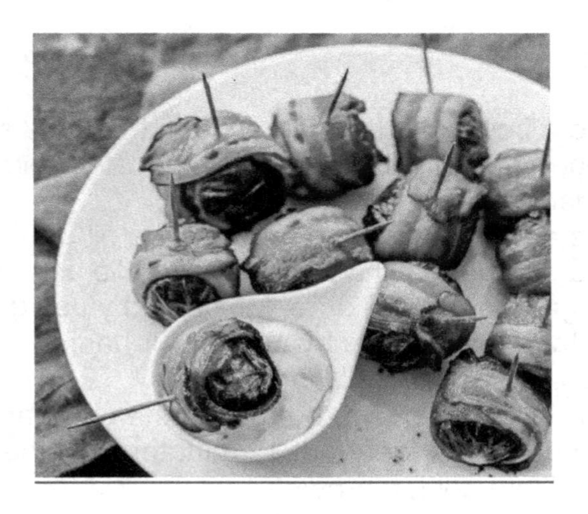

Preparing Time : 10 minutes
Cooking Time: 40 minutes
Servings: 4 people

Ingredients

- 13 slices of bacon
- 13 Brussels sprouts
- 5 tablespoons of mayonnaise
- 1 tablespoon of balsamic vinegar

Directions

- Preheat the oven at 400 degrees F lined with parchment paper and 13 toothpicks
- Wrap the Brussels sprouts and wrap then by using a toothpick and then place them in the baking sheet pan
- Bake them for about 40 minutes until they are tendered or turned into golden and crispy brown
- Now take a bowl add balsamic vinegar and mayonnaise mixture them well until well combined
- Serve them with the sauce and enjoy

Recipe No 39

Keto Turkey Bacon Ranch Pinwheels

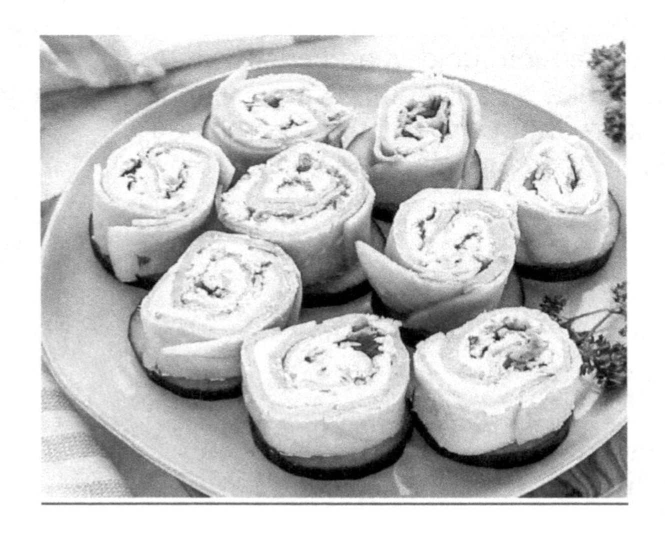

Preparing Time : 10 minutes
Cooking Time: 5 minutes
Servings: 6 people

Ingredients

- 6 ounces of cream cheese
- 12 slices of smoked deli turkey
- ¼ teaspoon of garlic powder
- ¼ teaspoon of dried minced onion
- 3 tablespoons of shredded mozzarella cheese
- 2 tablespoons of bacon crumbles

Directions

- Take 2 plastic wraps and place the cream cheese in between them.
- After that remove the top side of the plastic wrap them hold or lay the slices of turkey on the outer side of the cream cheese
- Then cover them with a new plastic wrap and cover the whole thing over. After sometime peel off the plastic wrap. Sprinkle some spices on them then sprinkle with some bacon and cheese
- Roll the turkey on the outside. Refrigerate them for 2 hours then serve them with the sliced cucumbers
- Enjoy

Recipe No 40

Smoked Trout Mousse

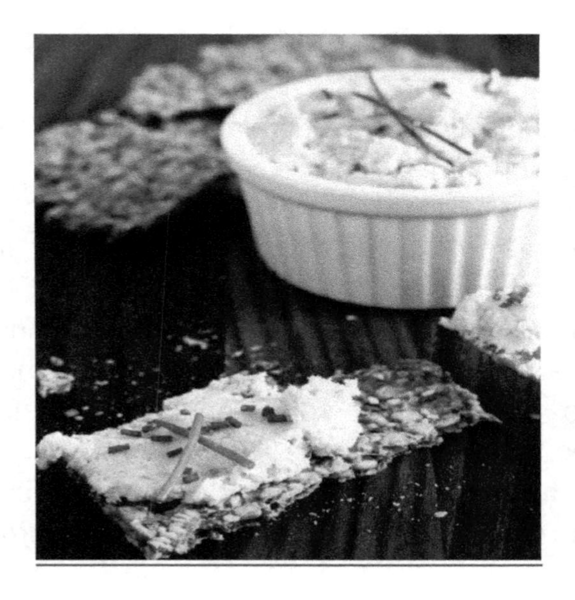

Preparing Time : 10 minutes
Cooking Time: 10 minutes
Servings: 8 people

Ingredients

- 10 ounces of smoked trout
- 2 cup of unsalted butter (softened)
- 2 tablespoons of horseradish
- 3 tablespoons of whipping cream
- 2 tablespoons of lemon juice
- Some kosher salt to taste
- Some ground white pepper to taste
- Some fresh chives finely chopped

Directions

- Take a food processor and add the smoked trout and process them for about 15 seconds
- After that add the butter and pulse them for more 15 seconds
- Then add the whipping cream, horseradish and other seasonings and pulse them until it is blended for 20 seconds
- Then taste them and add lemon juice and serve

Recipe No 41

Shrimp Rangoon Mini Bell Peppers Appetizer

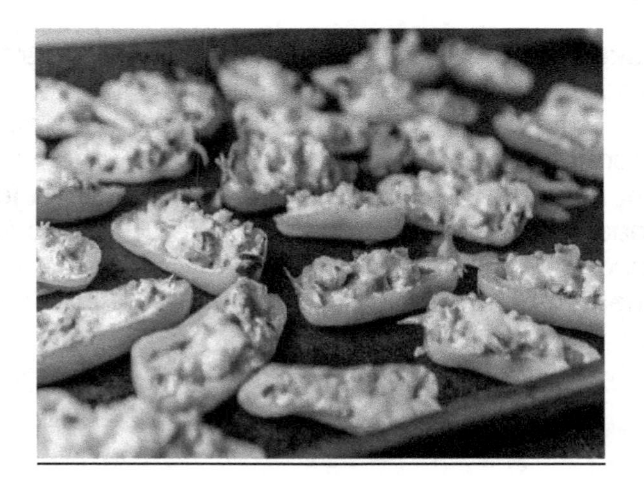

Preparing Time : 30 minutes
Cooking Time: 10 minutes
Servings: 6 people

Ingredients

- 20 bell peppers cut in half-sized then seeds removed
- ½ lbs of shrimps peeled and ends trimmed
- 1 teaspoon of chilli powder
- ½ teaspoon of garlic powder
- Some salt to taste
- 1 tablespoon of extra virgin olive oil
- 4 ounces of cream cheese softened
- 2 tablespoons of green onions thinly chopped
- 1 tablespoon of lemon juice
- ½ cup of shredded mozzarella cheese
- Some extra virgin olive oil for spraying

Directions

- Preheat the oven at 375 degrees F. Line the baking sheet with parchment paper and then spray with some extra virgin olive oil
- Take a bowl, add shrimps, salt, garlic powder and chilli powder to then combine them. Then take a nonstick pan and add olive oil and then cook the shrimps in them from both sides until it turns golden brown and crispy
- Then roughly chopped the cooked shrimps in a bowl
- Take another bowl add chopped shrimps, cream cheese, salt, like juice and green onions. Combine them well until all the ingredients are mixed together
- Take a baking sheet lined with parchment paper and sprayed with some olive oil put the bell peppers and fill them with cream cheese shrimps and then top them with shredded mozzarella cheese
- Bake them for about 10 minutes
- Remove them from the heat and then let them cool
- Serve them and enjoy

Recipe No 42

Keto Cranberry Brie Bites

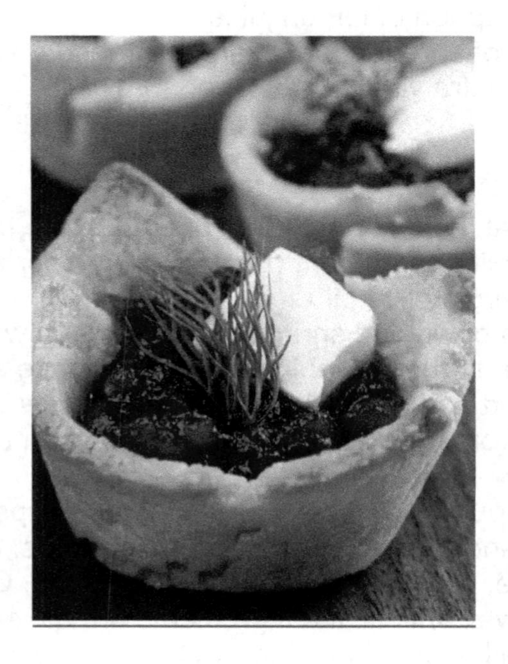

Preparing Time : 30 minutes
Cooking Time: 15 minutes
Servings: 6 people

Ingredients

For The Dough

- 2 cups of Mozzarella cheese
- 2 tablespoons of Almond butter
- 1 large golden Egg
- 1 teaspoon of Vanilla extract
- 1 cup of Almond flour
- ¼ teaspoon of Powdered stevia
- ½ teaspoon of Baking powder

For the Filling

- 4 tablespoons of cranberry sauce
- 3 ounces of brie cheese

Directions

- Take a bowl add mozzarella cheese let them microwave for about 30 seconds and let them melt
- Take a separate bowl add almond flour, stevia and baking powder. Stir them to combine
- Now crack the egg in the cheese bowl and add almond butter stir then together with the help of wooden spoon to mix them
- Then add the dry ingredients in the cream cheese mixture and combine them
- Make dough balls and putt then on the baking sheet and roll them to make them thick sheets
- Cut the dough in square shapes
- Then set them in a muffin silicone cup tray
- Bake them for about 5 minutes
- Then remove them from the oven and add the cranberry sauce and putting brie slices
- Again bake them for 7 minutes
- Serve them and enjoy

Recipe No 43

Keto Bacon, Egg And Cheese Slider Appetizer

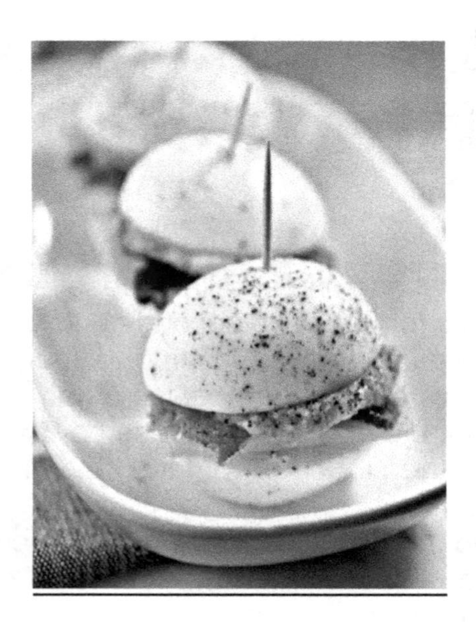

Preparing Time : 10 minutes
Cooking Time: 10 minutes
Servings: 6 people

Ingredients

- 6 golden eggs peeled and cut in half sized
- ½ avocado mashed
- 6 small slices of cheddar cheese
- 6 small slices of cooked bacon
- ½ tablespoon of lemon juice
- ½ teaspoon of cumin powder
- Some toothpicks as desired
- Some kosher salt to taste
- Some ground black pepper to taste

Directions

- Take a food processor, add avocado, lemon juice, some salt and black pepper. Blend them until well combined and smooth creamy batter is formed
- Take a plate and put the half cut sized eggs, place the cheese slice on them, then put the cooked bacon slices on them
- Then put the mashed avocado on the top
- Then put the other half size of the egg in the top and make a sandwich. Secure then by placing a toothpick in them
- Serve then and enjoy

Recipe No 44

Keto Ranch Dip

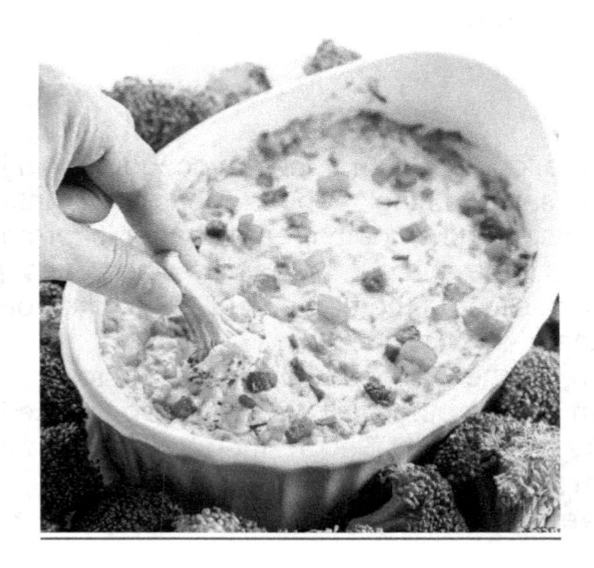

Preparing Time : 10 minutes
Cooking Time: 15 minutes
Servings: 15 people

Ingredients

- 2 cups of cream cheese
- ¾ cup of ranch dressing
- 4 tablespoons of sour cream
- 1 cup of shredded mozzarella cheese
- ⅓ cup of cooked bacon in bite-sized
- ⅓ cup of chopped green onions
- Pinch of cayenne pepper

Direction's

- Preheat the oven at 375 degrees F
- Take a bowl add the cream cheese mixture and microwave them for about 30 seconds
- Then add the sour cream and ranch dressing stir them to combine well
- Transfer the dip in the baking dish pan
- Bake them for about 15 minutes
- Serve them hot with veggies

Recipe No 45

Keto Shrimp Avocado Cucumber Bites

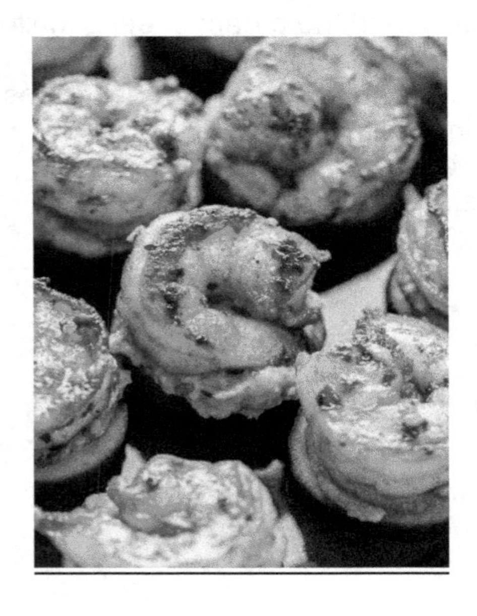

Preparing Time : 15 minutes
Cooking Time: 5 minutes
Servings: 22 people

Ingredients

- 1 lbs of shrimp peeled and ends trimmed
- 2 cloves of minced garlic
- 1 tablespoon of freshly chopped cilantro
- 1 teaspoon of paprika powder
- 1 teaspoon of cayenne pepper
- Some kosher salt to taste
- Some ground black pepper to taste
- 2 tablespoons of extra virgin olive oil

Avocado Spread

- 1 avocado mashed
- 1 tablespoon of lemon juice
- Some kosher salt to taste
- 1 large cucumber sliced

Directions

- Take a bowl, add shrimps, then add cayenne pepper, salt, pepper, minced garlic, cilantro, paprika powder, black pepper and olive oil. Toss them to coat well
- Take a nonstick skillet add the olive oil and put the shrimps cook them for about 2-3 minutes per side until it is cooked thoroughly
- Take another bowl add mashed avocados, some salt and lemon juice stir them to combine all the ingredients together
- Take the cucumber slices, put the mashed avocados and then put the shrimps. Sprinkle some chopped parsley and then serve them
- Enjoy

Recipe No 46

Salami Appetizers

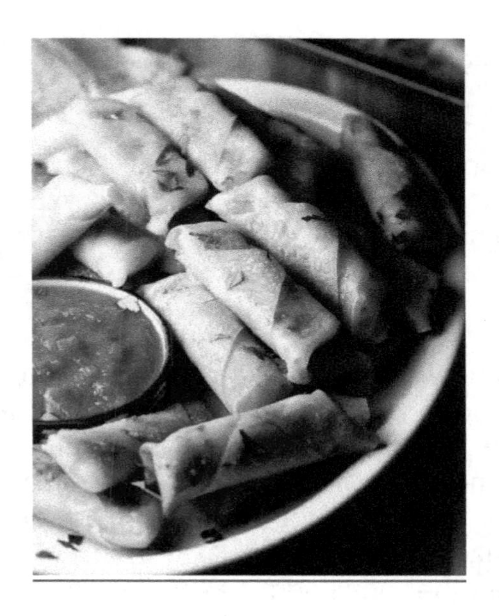

Preparing Time : 15 minutes
Cooking Time: 20 minutes
Servings: 32 bites

Ingredients

- 8 sticks of mozzarella cheese (cut them in lengthwise and then cut them half again)
- 32 squares of the wonton wrappers
- 32 rounds of salami
- Some extra virgin olive oil
- Freshly chopped parsley for garnishing
- Pizza sauce, marina sauce and spaghetti sauce for dipping

Directions

- Preheat the oven at 400 degrees F
- Line the baking pan with parchment paper
- Take a wonton wrapper and then place a piece of salami at the bottom of the wrapper. Then put the piece of cheese on top of the wrapper
- By folding of the both corners wrap them tightly by keeping it carefully so that the cheese shouldn't be leaked out. Seal it's corner by using water
- Repeat this process with the rest of the wrappers
- Bake them for about 15 minutes until it turns golden brown and then again bake them for an additional 5 minutes
- Remove them in a plate and then serve them with your favorite dipping sauce and enjoy

Recipe No 47

Keto Shrimp Guacamole

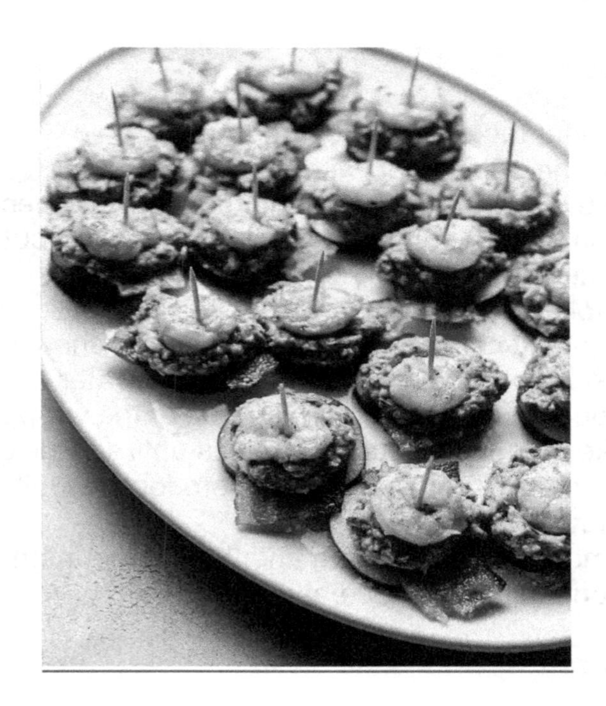

Preparing Time : 20 minutes
Cooking Time: 20 minutes
Servings: 20 people

Ingredients

Guacamole

- 2 avocados
- ½ cup of minced red onion
- 1 tablespoon of lemon juice
- ½ cup of fresh cilantro lightly packed
- Some kosher salt to taste

Shrimps

- 20 shrimps peeled and deveined
- Some kosher salt to taste
- Some ground black pepper
- ¼ teaspoon of cumin powder
- 2 tablespoons of butter

Other Ingredients

- 7 slices of bacon cooked and crisped (cut into thirds)
- 1 large cucumber cut into thin slices

Directions

- Take a food processor and add all the guacamole ingredients in the and process them until well combined
- Take a bowl add shrimps, salt, pepper and cumin powder toss them until they are well combined and coated
- Take a nonstick pan, add butter, let them what and then add the shrimps. Cook them from both sides until they are fully cooked
- Now take a plate and lay down the slices of cucumber. Put in them bacon then guacamole and then top them with the shrimp
- Serve them and enjoy

Recipe No 48

Keto Cranberry Meatballs

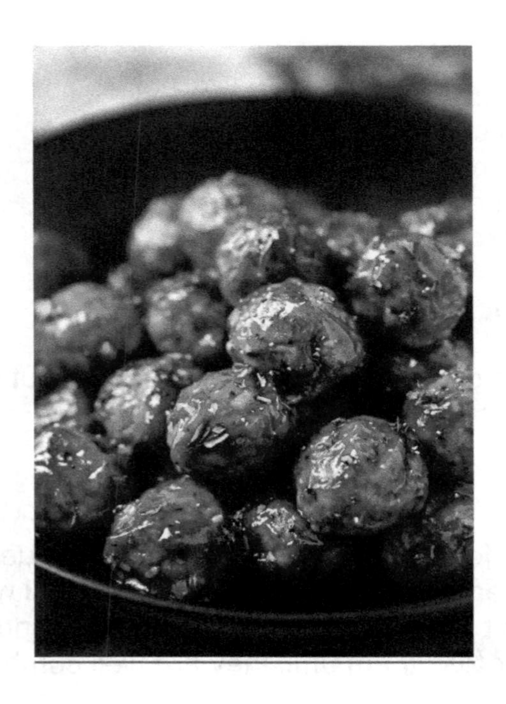

Preparing Time : 5 minutes
Cooking Time: 3 hours
Servings: 14 people

Ingredients

- 60 frozen meatballs
- 20 ounces bottle of BBQ sauce
- 12 ounces can of jellied cranberry sauce
- Freshly chopped parsley to garnish
- Some kosher salt to taste
- Some ground black pepper to taste

Directions

- Take a bowl, add BBQ sauce and jellied cranberry sauce. Stir them to combine well
- Take a slow cooker, add meatballs and then drizzle the sauce. Cook then on low flame for about 3 hours
- After that time pour them in a bowl and garnish with finely chopped parsley and serve them
- Enjoy

Recipe No 49

Sour Cream And Onion Keto Chips

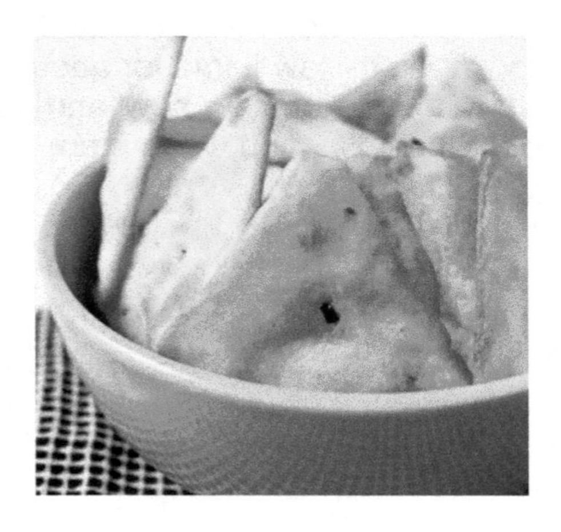

Preparing Time : 15 minutes
Cooking Time: 10 minutes
Servings: 4 people

Ingredients

- 2 cups of shredded mozzarella cheese
- 2 tablespoons of butter
- 1 golden egg
- 2 tablespoons of sour cream
- ¾ cup of almond flour
- ½ teaspoon of onion powder
- ½ teaspoon of garlic powder
- ½ teaspoon of mustard powder
- Some kosher salt to taste
- Some chopped chives

Directions

- Preheat the oven at 375 degrees F
- Prepare the baking sheet lined with parchment paper
- Take an ovenproof bowl and add mozzarella cheese and butter. Melt them for 2 minutes until it is softened
- Then remove them from the oven and add sour cream and egg beat them with an electric beater
- Then add the almond flour, garlic powder, onion powder, mustard powder and salt. Mix all the ingredients together until thick dough is formed
- Mix the chives in the dough and then knead them. Place them in the refrigerator to settle
- Then take out the dough and knead them until it turns in a very thin layer
- Peel the dough in triangular form and then place them on the baking pan lined with parchment paper
- Place them in the baking oven for about 10 minutes until it turns golden brown and crispy
- Then serve them with your favorite sauce and enjoy

Recipe No 50

Keto Zucchini Pizza Crust

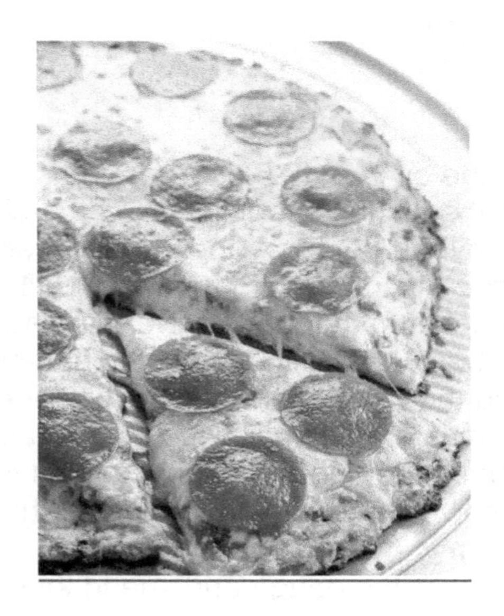

Preparing Time : 15 minutes
Cooking Time: 30 minutes
Servings: 8 people

Ingredients

- 8 ounces of grated zucchini
- 3 large golden eggs
- 1 cup of shredded mozzarella cheese
- 4 tablespoons of coconut flour
- Some sea salt to taste
- Some thinly sliced pepperonis

Directions

- Preheat the oven at 37t degrees F
- Take a nonstick baking tray oil lined with parchment paper greased with some oil
- Take a bowl add the grated zucchini and squeeze them to remove the excess moisture then add some salt and stir them to combine
- Spread this grated zucchini in the pan evenly and bake them for 15 minutes until it is soft
- Till then take a bowl and mozzarella cheese, salt, coconut flour, and eggs. Whisk them together until well combined
- Check the zucchini if it's done then pat dry with a paper towel
- Remove the pan from the oven and then mix them zucchini in the egg bowl and mix all the ingredients together until well combined and thick pizza dough is formed
- Place them in the parchment lined pizza pan and then spread the crust in the pan and then let them bake for about 10 minutes
- Then remove the pan and sprinkle some grated cheddar cheese and pepperoni slices
- Bake them for about 10 minutes until the cheese is melted
- Serve them with your favorite sauce and enjoy

Notes

CPSIA information can be obtained
at www.ICGtesting.com
Printed in the USA
LVHW080743050521
686549LV00005B/230